TESTIM<

I have seen, first hand, many instances where children and families have been totally transformed by addressing food sensitivities, If you suspect food may be the cause of your child's physical and behavioral symptoms, you must read this well researched and practical approach to discovering your particular child's trigger food(s) and developing a plan to address them. Margaret Evans offers hope in this clearly presented and easily read book. Read it. It could positively change your child's and family's lives.

Fran Richardson RN BscN (retired) Pediatric Nurse

Through many years of dedicated work and practice, Margaret Evans has developed an incredibly informative and useful guide for all those suffering from food related symptoms. Intelligent, comprehensive and most importantly, do-able, her supportive and effective direction was an essential component on my path towards optimum health.

Meghan MacCallum, Age 29

"Daniel is a wonderful four year old, but much of a challenge. The change we have seen in him since altering his diet, I could not have imagined would be possible. My only regret is that we did not contact Margaret earlier. We are now a happy, healthy family with sane parents! I cannot recommend her more highly."

Sarah, Richard, and Daniel Jones

Since I was little I have had stomach aches, exhaustion, nightmares, IBS and many other symptoms. I found hope and answers to my struggles when I met Margaret. By removing dairy and gluten products from my diet I am now healthy, full of life, and enjoying the two children we were able to conceive. Both our children are thriving and healthy on a dairy and gluten free diet, as well. Margaret has been such a blessing.

Ashlyn Faber, 24 years old

Knowledgeable, timely, and practical! Margaret's advice and encouragement during our family's transition to a gluten-free, dairy-free way of life kept us on track, motivated to persevere, and thankful for the remarkable improvements we've experienced. A health concern for one family member has turned into life-long benefits for six! Thanks, Margaret!

A grateful grandmother

As a Registered Nurse I thought I understood nutrition and its impact on the body. Not so! After listening to Margaret Evans explain about food intolerances I learned a lot and realized that my son's symptoms fit right into what she was saying. I had a much healthier and happier son when dairy products were removed from his diet. Thank you so much Margaret for your help with my son's diet and health and mine as well.

Margaret Kerr R.N., B.S.N.

One of the most significant changes I made in my life as a result of coaching with Marg was changing my family's eating habits. Many symptoms and behaviors that had been problems for years with my children disappeared! After we were successful with the food sensitivities, I knew that the rest of my life was going to change—for the better! I can hardly imagine how alone in the world I felt, before meeting Margaret.

Tina Meyer

Initially, I was not a believer that food could have such a powerful impact on one's health and function. By age four, my son was still not sleeping through the night, had a runny nose and tummy aches. My daughter had frequent digestion issues that interfered with her daily life. After learning about food sensitivities through Margaret, I was able to successfully identify and eliminate the correct foods the correct way. To my delight and surprise within 3 weeks all of my children's issues completely disappeared. Today, our family eats a wider variety of foods than before, rarely get sick and experiences greater overall health and vitality.

L. North

After enduring many months of low energy, joint pain and numerous other undiagnosed ailments, I was struggling in all areas of life but particularly in my role of helping others. I was amazed and relieved to finally discover that culprit foods were the reason for my symptoms. When I stopped eating these foods, my recovery was remarkable. I am so thankful for the wisdom and practical methods that Margaret has shared with me, allowing me to live well with my food sensitivities and to offer hope and understanding to my clients.

**Karen Sollid BSc(Nutr) RD Registered Dietitian
and Certified Wellness Coach**

Margaret Evans has been teaching at the Boucher Institute of Naturopathic Medicine for several years now and is considered the leader in food sensitivity diagnosis and treatment. Evans has given us a much-needed step-by-step guide to truly finding and dealing with foods allergies and the health problems they cause. We in the practice of Naturopathic medicine are grateful for this much anticipated work.

**Anders B. Nerman (Naturopathic Student) Boucher Institute
of Naturopathic Medicine Vancouver BC Canada**

Margaret Evans offers a thorough, compassionate inquiry into the deep threads of a patient's diet and lifestyle which may be holding them back from their potential. Her 30+ years of clinical experience along with her extensive knowledge has allowed Margaret to find her own approach which is empowering yet healing for her clients. She lives her work and provides healthcare professionals with the inspiration to spend the time to find the cause of their patient's limitations. Thank you Margaret, my approach to patients has changed!

**Karley Denoon (Naturopathic Student) Boucher Institute
of Naturopathic Medicine, Vancouver, B.C. Canada**

Could It Really Be Something They Ate?

The Life Changing Impact of Addressing Food Sensitivities in Children

Margaret Evans, RN, BScN, CPCC

BALBOA.
PRESS

A DIVISION OF HAY HOUSE

Balboa Press books may be ordered through booksellers or by contacting:

Balboa Press
A Division of Hay House
1663 Liberty Drive
Bloomington, IN 47403
www.balboapress.com
1-(877) 407-4847

ISBN: 978-1-4525-4159-4 (sc)
ISBN: 978-1-4525-4160-0 (hc)
ISBN: 978-1-4525-4158-7 (e)

Library of Congress Control Number: 2011919165

Because of the dynamic nature of the Internet, any web addresses or links contained in this book may have changed since publication and may no longer be valid. The views expressed in this work are solely those of the author and do not necessarily reflect the views of the publisher, and the publisher hereby disclaims any responsibility for them.

The author of this book does not dispense medical advice or prescribe the use of any technique as a form of treatment for physical, emotional, or medical problems without the advice of a physician, either directly or indirectly. The intent of the author is only to offer information of a general nature to help you in your quest for emotional and spiritual well-being. In the event you use any of the information in this book for yourself, which is your constitutional right, the author and the publisher assume no responsibility for your actions.

Photography: Bopomo Pictures
Graphic Illustration: Cliff Webb
Cover design: Chelsea Bell Eady

Printed in the United States of America

Balboa Press rev. date: 12/16/2011

DEDICATION

This book is dedicated to my husband, Ken, and
our four children, Rob, Cari, Steve, and Jodie,
in celebration of the love, support, patience,
and laughter we have offered each other in this
journey to find health.

"Hope Is the Anchor of the Soul"
(Hebrews 6:19)

ACKNOWLEDGMENTS

The journey of writing this book has allowed me to reminisce and celebrate the many people who have touched my life. My story is rich with both successes and disappointments, and every experience has taught me many valuable lessons. I would not have been able to write this book without them all.

To God—I am grateful for your unconditional love and continuous, unwavering support throughout my life. Your placement of that glowing book on the shelf in a Toronto bookstore almost thirty years ago began a journey of healing that I would never have imagined was possible. Although I initially thought I was hallucinating, it turned out that you had heard my prayers for help and offered me the book I needed to address the food sensitivities in our children. Our children would not be well and this book would not have been written without your graceful support.

To my parents who are no longer here—thank you for teaching me to persevere through adversity with the faith and trust that hope is always just around the corner. Your lessons of resilience in the face of challenges helped me keep going when things were difficult. Your unconditional love and support of Ken, me, and your grandchildren enabled you to embrace the many diet changes we made with grace and patience. Thank you for your love and acceptance.

To my husband, Ken—you have been my strength, my friend, and my biggest fan for over thirty-five years. Without your willingness to support me, our journey as a family, and my writing of this book, this story would never have been told. I love you.

To our children, Rob, Cari, Steve, and Jodie—you have been the guinea pigs of many of my ideas and have been more patient with it all than I could ever have imagined. You have always been my motivation to reach for more, try again, and believe that anything is possible. You are amazing adults, and I am proud of the wonderful people you have become.

To our daughter-in-law, Tanya, and son-in-law, Gordon—thank you for embracing this path of health along with our children. Adding you to our family has been a huge gift, and it is wonderful to watch the happiness you have brought to our children and the health you are nurturing in our grandchildren.

To our two little grandsons, Alex and Gabriel, and our new little granddaughter, Cameron—your health and love of life have allowed me to celebrate the impact of what I have learned in the last twenty five years. Your stories are different from our children's stories as babies and toddlers, and I am grateful for that. May you embrace the health your parents are modeling for you and carry that gift with you always. Nana and Granddad love you very much.

To my lifelong friends, Fran and Marg—you have listened patiently to the stories of my life and been there through it all. I have laughed, cried, celebrated, and mourned with you through a multitude of experiences. You have loved our kids through the many stages of their lives and felt like part of our family. I love you both and consider you wonderful blessings in my life.

To my many other wonderful friends—you know who you are. Some of you spent countless hours on the phone with me, planning menus for our kids' diets. Some of you sat in skating and hockey rinks, stood at field hockey sidelines, and participated in countless other activities with me as we supported each other's kids. Some of you listened and supported me when I was discouraged and unsure what direction to go and celebrated my successes. Some of you supported our kids when they needed the warm and accepting influence of other caring adults. It is the village you all created around me and my family that has made our journey so rich with memories. I am grateful to you all.

To the hundreds of families who have courageously shared their stories with me and allowed me to help them find the health and happiness they longed for—I am grateful for your vulnerability and trust. It is only by hearing your stories that I am able to write this book.

To Gordon, my wonderful editor—thank you. When God invited you into the story of my book, he offered me a huge gift. Your gentle and encouraging manner and constant reminders to listen and feel my way rather than push have made the writing of this book a wonderful experience. I look forward to a lifelong friendship from here.

To Cari, my proof reader extraordinaire—thank you for the time and special attention you gave to the final draft of my book despite nursing your newborn baby! The book is so much better because of your wonderful wisdom.

CONTENTS

FOREWORD

As a naturopathic physician and acupuncturist, I have witnessed a dramatic increase—especially over the past ten years—in the incidence of inflammatory and behavioral conditions in children, including eczema, asthma, allergies, ADHD, and autism. Of particular concern is the increase of such conditions in babies less than a year old. A massive and often overlooked underlying cause of these pediatric issues is adverse food reactions, also known as food sensitivities.

In *Could It Really Be Something They Ate?,* Margaret has compiled her incredible knowledge of food sensitivities in a book that is clearly written, readily accessible, and will be an invaluable resource to all parents whose children are struggling with symptoms potentially related to food.

I have had the pleasure of working closely with Margaret and appreciate the wisdom and expertise she offers to our patients. As a pediatric nurse with extensive nutrition experience, life coach, and mother of four children herself, Margaret has a wealth of experience related to food sensitivities. She has been a consultant to parents and children on food-triggered health concerns for over twenty-five years, with countless success stories of children's lives being dramatically improved—and even saved—under her caring guidance.

Current information about this common health issue is often confusing and misguided. There are many different restrictive elimination diets available that require the removal of multiple foods from a child's diet. The list of foods to avoid can be so long and varied that many parents are not able to sustain the change in diet. As a parent myself, I know firsthand how much work goes into providing a healthy, balanced diet for my children. Just thinking of removing several foods at once from my daughters' diets feels overwhelming. I have seen many parents who have given up evaluating food sensitivities in their children because the recommendations they received from a health care professional felt unsustainable.

Margaret uses an individualized and thorough approach to help parents determine their child's primary trigger food. This is done through a detailed health history questionnaire and symptom checklist. Her goal is to remove the least amount of foods (ideally just one) from the diet as possible while allowing for maximal improvement in children's health. Although conventional and alternative food sensitivity tests are often helpful, it is possible that their results will actually miss the main trigger food. When this happens, even the elimination of multiple foods results in very little symptom improvement. The common-sense approach described in this book will help prevent this unfortunate oversight from occurring.

After detailing her approach for trigger food identification, Margaret shares practical ways for parents to undertake changes in their child's diet. While acknowledging the challenges parents often face with this process, she dispels many common myths about elimination diets for children and provides real-world, attainable options for successfully addressing their food sensitivities. A lack of preparation is a major reason for failure, and Margaret dedicates an entire chapter to a self-evaluation process parents can complete before they begin removing the offending food from their child's diet. Children can have significant emotional reactions to changes in their typical diet, including tears, tantrums, and cravings. The reasons for them and effective coping strategies for parents are described in great detail. Margaret finishes by sharing her own amazing personal health history that led to the writing of this book and the fulfilling work that she does.

As one who has witnessed firsthand the life-changing results of her work, it gives me great personal satisfaction to know this book will expand the reach of Margaret's life-changing work far beyond her busy consulting practice.

And yes, I can wholeheartedly say to you—It really *could* be something they ate!

Dr. Arjuna Veeravagu
Naturopathic Physician and Registered Acupuncturist
Sage Clinic
Vancouver, British Columbia
Canada

INTRODUCTION

Experience, Strength, and Hope

Most people I know have a personal love affair with cheese—grilled in a panini, creamed in a fabulous dessert, or just a slice straight from the fridge. What is it about cheese that is so unbelievably delicious? My own inclinations to eat cheese at every meal are no different, but I have a food sensitivity to dairy that makes me feel horrible if I eat even a little! Most people I know could not imagine giving up a food that they eat in such abundance and find so tempting. Most people I know find that they have strong willpower for other decisions and disciplines in their lives but have a very challenging time when it comes to food.

So how do I get a handle on what I eat and stay motivated enough to keep away from the cheese? For me, it is about prioritizing. Experience has taught me that what I eat has as much—and sometimes more—impact on my health as the amount of sleep I get, the decisions I make at work, and the way I monitor my relationships and emotions. It has a profound impact on the overall stress level of my life. My health is invaluable to me, and with the help of my mom, I have learned some important lessons over the last thirty years about how to keep myself healthy, happy, and full of energy rather than succumbing to stomach aches, moodiness, and exhaustion.

I came by two values very honestly in my life: a focus on health and a determination to figure out solutions to challenges. As a young child,

I was a delightful baby who suddenly became a terror at two. I would not sleep, screamed all the time at the drop of a hat, and had constant tummy aches and diarrhea. I flung myself into dramatic tantrums—both at home and in public. What had happened to my mom's happy and content little girl? Beyond dealing with my behavior, my mom had to deal with the skepticism of others when she insisted to friends and to people in the medical community that my behavior was not just a case of the terrible twos. My mother taught me that little kids are supposed to be naturally happy, content, and healthy. She fought for me when others would have given up. She kept reading, asking, researching, and persisting, and eventually learned about food sensitivities.

My mom discovered that these new health and behavior challenges of mine were a result of food sensitivities to dairy and eggs. She looks back now at pictures of me eating grilled cheese sandwiches and egg laden angel food cake with seven-minute frosting and shivers, knowing those foods were what triggered these difficult changes. Growing up, I never really felt that different because of my food sensitivities; in my family, we all had certain things we didn't eat, and it was just a way of life. Having to avoid dairy and eggs was much the same for me as having to clean my room or bring the laundry up from the basement: it was a household expectation, and I just did it. It rarely seemed a hardship—I remember my mom going out of her way to ensure that there was always delicious food to eat. She baked constantly, usually two versions of the same muffins (one egg and dairy-free for me and one-gluten-free for my brother and sister) and always had delicious, kid-friendly snacks around the house.

The Evans' place was known as a great spot to come and eat by our friends. Outside our house, it was no different; my mom still went the extra mile. I remember her coming to my elementary school with a McDonald's hamburger and fries when the hot dogs at hot dog day contained something I couldn't eat; I remember her making me a cake so that I could bring my own *huge* slice to a birthday party I was invited to. I was not left out, as there was always something tasty to replace what I could not eat.

Did I stay 100 percent egg and dairy free throughout elementary and high school? No, but I still remember the disappointed faces of my parents when I cheated. My knowledge of their disappointment, combined with the fact that I did not physically feel well, was a strong deterrent. Disappointing them by eating something unhealthy for me was the same as disappointing them by lying to them or saying something mean to one of my siblings.

I don't think any child grows up without testing their parents' boundaries, but I do think that the consistency of parental expectations is integral to setting a standard they will return to. My parents treated our eating habits much the same way as they treated other values of our family, such as avoiding alcohol and drugs. The expectation was just that you did not do them, and that expectation was never compromised.

As a teacher, I understand the importance of modeling that same consistency in my classroom. If my students are allowed to do something one day and not the next, they become confused and have a difficult time discerning my expectations. If I truly do not want them to exhibit some behavior or way of treating others, I need to be consistent in my expectations and clear in my expression of them. It is my parents' modeling of this consistency of expectations that taught me the importance of being true to my health, and it is a lifelong lesson that has carried over into adulthood.

As an adult, I have come to understand food sensitivities and healthy eating habits in a much more detailed way. I am aware that eating a variety of different kinds of fruits, grains, and vegetables is important. I also know that my body reacts differently during times of stress, and that I need to adjust my eating habits accordingly. Some foods I rotate through my regular diet are generally fine for my system, but aggravate me in the times when I am low on sleep, feel the frantic pace of life, or am getting a cold, for example. These times of high stress are when, I know from experience, to also not eat tomatoes and soy so my body has the best chance possible to recuperate its immune system.

How many people get sick on a regular basis and think nothing of it because it is such a constant in their lives? I am grateful that I have learned ways to help myself stay as healthy as I can. The challenging part is that I have to do more than just know what foods to stay away from. I read labels to be aware of ingredients, know how to bake by replacing eggs with other substitutes, make time to cook tasty meals at home, look up menus online before going to dinner at new restaurants, and plan ahead to have healthy food that I can eat when I go away for a weekend. The most important part for me is that I have to be willing to put the time into making sure that I am eating food that is satisfying and interesting so that I continue to love eating healthy. When you eat foods that taste good and that you love, you don't feel deprived or resentful, and staying on a healthy regimen is much easier.

Besides surrounding myself with tasty food, I find surrounding myself with people who are respectful of my food sensitivities to be another key to staying healthy. To me, someone who respects and supports your decisions is just a good friend, whether that friend is supporting your wish to not eat dairy, be vegetarian, dye your hair red, not have any children, or save money by staying on a budget. Eating within my food sensitivities is just one way I make decisions in my life that are right for me. Staying true to my choice of avoiding dairy and eggs is the same to me as the other values that I honor in my life. I have no doubt that this strength of character and belief in doing what is right for me was intentionally cultivated by my parents as I was growing up. Their message was always to not compromise what is important. My health is important to me, and I make choices in my life to support that ideal.

As I now navigate the first few months of parenthood, I am more aware of my health and what I eat than ever before. My health and thus my daughter's health directly affect the level of stress in our home. As my husband and I continue to learn how much work is involved in being parents, we cannot imagine having more than the usual challenges (and less than the usual amount of sleep!) with a newborn. We are grateful to have been proactive in our decision for me to eat a healthy diet and conscientiously avoid the foods to which I am intolerant, and have focused on making both my pregnancy and time breastfeeding as positive and healthy as possible. I have heard stories of the challenges that my siblings and I experienced as babies and toddlers and have no idea how my mom survived! At a time when so much is new and out of our control, my husband and I are grateful to have one less thing to worry about. Our daughter is healthy and thriving and, unlike many babies, does not have colic, ear infections, green poop, or a chronic runny nose. This is one of the times in my life when I have, without a doubt, had the most motivation to stay on my diet.

My experience with parenthood, however, is not the first time in my life when food and health have taken on a specifically important meaning. Training to run a marathon, managing time and stress while planning a wedding, and dealing with a changing metabolism at the age of thirty all caused me to pay special attention to the foods I was eating. I have learned that when my awareness of health is heightened to focus on achieving a specific goal, there are more benefits than just the absence of stomach aches. I treat other people with more patience, have a more positive attitude, need less sleep, have a stronger immune system, and am more physically fit. Learning about food sensitivities has helped me to learn many other things about healthy eating that I also try to integrate into my life. Most people in my life do not know me as someone who eats a dairy and egg-free diet; they know me as someone who tries to maintain healthy eating habits, loves to cook—and most importantly, as someone who loves to eat! Staying true to my food sensitivity diet is about more than just feeling good physically; it is about creating and continuing a healthy and happy lifestyle that helps me fulfill my potential and use my personality strengths to the best of my ability.

I believe every human being possesses amazing potential and that often all we need to help us reach this potential is to change certain habits. Changing one's habits is powerful—we just need the right understanding and motivation to do it. As a high school teacher, I know that teenagers need support to help them through change, and adults are no different. I had strong family support when my diet was changed as a child, and I now have a wonderful husband and community of friends who respect and encourage the choices I make for my own health and my own life.

One of the most powerful realizations for me has been that once my habits are truly in place, they rarely waver. When my life gets difficult, I have the tools to know what to do. No matter what the change—whether living through the stress of studying for university exams or settling myself to live and work in a different country—I return to eating what is best for my health because I know it works and never fails to sustain me.

I am grateful that my parents taught me about self-care and independence, that my mom fought to find a solution that has allowed me to live a full and amazing life, and that both my parents set such a strong example of character and consistency. Food sensitivities have always been a prevalent topic in my life, but they have set the stage for me to develop knowledge of myself and strength of character that goes far beyond the food I eat.

These choices are about the food, and yet, are about vastly more than that. To me, it is really about choosing how you want to live your life and loving the life you've chosen to live.

Cari Evans, B.A., B. Educ.
Vancouver, British Columbia

PREFACE

What we call despair is often only the painful eagerness
of unfed hope.
George Eliot

Twenty-five years ago, I was a worried and overwhelmed mom of three children under the age of five. Despite my years as a pediatric nurse and my husband's training as a physician, we seemed unable to find answers to the health, behavior, and learning challenges of our children. The stomach aches, fatigue, chronic diarrhea, multiple ear infections, bladder inflammation, and constant tantrums were exhausting to both my husband and me. Despite appointments with multiple specialists, we were unable to find any answers, and we felt lost and frustrated. A chance encounter in a bookstore twenty-five years ago addressing the topic of food sensitivities changed everything.

Today, the story of our family is very different. We have four adult children, a son-in-law, a daughter-in-law, and three grandchildren, and all are healthy and thriving. By addressing food sensitivities early in their lives, I transformed the direction and the potential of our children's futures. As a nurse and life coach, I have had the privilege of improving the health, behavior, and learning of hundreds of other children and their families. It is immensely rewarding work and the motivator behind the writing of this book.

Why would we consider changing the diets of our children to try and eliminate a few troublesome symptoms? Most of us as parents are already busy and stretched to the limit. Why not just accept their symptoms as normal and simply find a medication that will improve them? For me, the answer to this question is clear—as parents, we are charged with the responsibility of helping our children be the best they can be. It is not about making them smarter than the neighbor's child or more successful so we look good. It is about supporting who they are and who they are meant to be. It is about helping them realize their full potential. By doing all we can to improve their health and embrace a healthy way of living during their childhood, we offer them the best chance of sustaining these practices into adulthood.

I see children every day who are suffering under the symptoms that can be created by food. They may be exhibiting behavior that results in them being ostracized by their peers. It may be that their health issues are so severe, they are unable to participate in sports or go to camp with their friends. They may be facing the challenges of obesity and feel like failures as they struggle over and over to stay off junk food but just can't seem to do it. It might be that learning is so difficult they have given up working toward careers they had hoped to achieve. It may also be that their families are so stressed by the situations these challenges create that everyone is in a state of turmoil, frustration, and constant irritation. Marriages often fall apart, and children suffer when families are overwhelmed with stress and worry. These examples are all true, and I have hundreds more.

According to the American Centre for Disease Control and Prevention, obesity in school aged children has risen from four percent in the early 1970's to 19.6 percent in 2008.[1] Asthma and autism are on the increase as well. As families spread out and relatives are less available to offer support, many of today's families feel overwhelmed. With more parents working full-time, the balancing act of raising a family is increasingly challenging. Finding time to address the diet and overall health concerns of their children can be frustrating and difficult. Many families are doing the very best they can, but when their children's health seems to be deteriorating, they struggle to figure out what to do. The solutions they are able to find often focus on short term fixes rather than long term, sustainable changes.

I have seen many families whose children are struggling, and the parents are at the end of their rope. They may have seen a number of health care professionals and come away feeling more overwhelmed than before. The diet changes to address food sensitivities may be confusing, and even physicians who offer help in this area may be unaware of the real-life challenges faced in implementing the recommendations they have suggested. Well-meaning and caring parents give the diet a try but very often abandon the process before discovering if food is the cause of their child's problems. Addressing the diet of their child is forgotten, and they may move on to look for other solutions or accept their child's situation as hopeless.

For all of us, change is edgy and difficult, and we often resist it. I have personally struggled through many situations where the idea of baking a different muffin seemed like too much bother, and the time it took to create a dinner that addressed everyone's needs seemed overwhelming. I have lived these stories over and over myself and have watched others do the same. I can also testify, however, to the amazing difference a diet change can make.

This book is based on a unique philosophy and process I have developed over my twenty-five years of working in the area of food sensitivities. I believe the topic is important for families to consider, and I have been committed to creating a process that is simple, successful, and that addresses the balance and complexities of a family's real life. By identifying a single trigger food and removing only this food for a month, the child's health often improves dramatically. It is not necessary to remove multiple foods that result in parents finding it almost impossible to create appealing school lunches or take their child out to dinner. By rotating the other foods in their family's diet and replacing the food that was removed with a healthy, age-appropriate alternative, children move closer and closer to a healthy and balanced diet, and the quality of their lives improve.

When children are regularly consuming the trigger food that is the cause of their symptoms, it results in their diets becoming increasingly limited, and attempts at expanding their food choices are often met with huge resistance. This is also the reason that children struggling with obesity find it almost impossible to eliminate high-fat and high-calorie junk foods. If their trigger food is dairy products, for example, they are so addicted to these foods that temporary and intermittent removal makes them crave these foods even more. Only by removing the trigger food 100 percent for a month can children be relieved of these cravings and find their way back to a healthy and balanced diet.

This book offers real solutions and real support for real families. If you have been to a health care professional or considered the idea of addressing your child's diet on your own but felt intimidated by the concept, relax and read this book. It is written in a format that is user-friendly and allows you to pick a small section and read even just a page or two. All of us are busy, and perhaps you only have time to read the summary at the end of a chapter. That is a great beginning, too. In the end, for all of us, change is about motivation. We can always find time to do what we believe is important. There are many parts of this book to help you find this motivation as well as support to address the other complex aspects of your life that might get in the way of your success. This book even offers some child and parent-friendly menu ideas to help you get going.

I believe, wholeheartedly, that successful change is only possible when a holistic approach is taken. Only by taking stock of all the aspects of your life will you be able to find your way to sustainable change. Finding the commitment and perseverance to change your child's diet may be the missing piece to allow their full potential to be realized. I can still remember the phone call I received from our daughter's junior kindergarten teacher two weeks after I adjusted the diet of our family. The teacher called to inquire what I had done to transform our daughter.

She had gone, in two weeks, from a tired, cranky little girl with tummy aches to a bright, inquisitive, energetic child who loved school and life. She remains that way to this day, twenty-six years later.

I know that we all connect best to stories, so my book is full of them, with only the names and situations changed to protect my client's anonymity. I hope, as you read these stories, you will find pieces of your own experience. I also hope you will be able to find the motivation to take a chance and address the diet of *your* family. As I watch our energetic and healthy grandchildren enjoy life to the fullest, I can remember back to the struggles our children had at the same age. I have not only changed the health of our children, but also of the next generation. There is nothing in this world that brings me more joy.

It is my dream that as you read and work through *Could It Really Be Something They Ate?* you will discover a sense of hope—hope for your child and hope for yourself. Perhaps the answers to some of your children's challenges will be found by addressing the issue of food sensitivities. I encourage you to consider the possibility. Perhaps the health of your child and the joy of your family will be transformed—just as ours was.

CHAPTER ONE

HOW DO I KNOW IF FOOD IS THE PROBLEM?

How do you know if the symptoms your child is experiencing are related to food? Are they just typical symptoms that most children experience, or are there problems you should be worried about? Is this just a stage that your child will outgrow, or will it create a problem for them in later years? In this chapter, you will find the answer to these questions. The symptoms that can potentially be related to food are varied and involve almost any part of the body. You will find some stories of typical clients of mine that demonstrate both the physical and emotional implications of eating foods that are problematic for an individual child. You will then find a detailed checklist of the signs and symptoms potentially related to food to complete for your own child. If you find yourself ticking multiple symptoms or several symptoms within one body system, the chances are very high that food is contributing to your child's health, behavior, or learning challenges.

In chapter three, you will then complete an additional questionnaire to determine the food that is the most likely cause or trigger of your child's symptoms. Rather than remove multiple foods or expose your child to a multitude of unpleasant tests, this process will help you pinpoint the cause of your child's symptoms. The remainder of the book then leads you, step by step, through the process to make the diet changes successfully.

REAL-LIFE STORIES

The combination of symptoms that can appear in one individual varies widely. These stories are based on clients I have worked with and demonstrate the wide range of symptoms that can be caused by a food as well as the dramatic impact these symptoms can have on the life of a child and their family.

Johnny, age two: colic as a baby, eczema, asthma, chronic ear infections, red and itchy penis, and chronic diarrhea.

Jodie can't believe how exhausted she is caring for her two-year-old son, Johnny. She barely has time to exercise and finds herself resorting often to quick snacks of yogurt, cheese and crackers. She knew motherhood would be busy, but she never imagined how many unexpected things would appear. Johnny seemed to cry from the moment he was born and was inconsolable much of the time. As a baby, he slept for only thirty minutes at a time, and now, even at the age of two, wakes up at least four times a night. Johnny was breastfed for the first six months, and then Jodie switched to soya formula in a desperate attempt to improve Johnny's colic and the eczema that had appeared on the soles of his feet and on his cheeks. From the age of six months on, Johnny's eczema and colic improved on the new soya formula, only to be replaced by chronic ear infections and a red, irritated rash at the end of his penis. For each ear infection, Johnny had a weeklong course of antibiotics, and over the next few months, each course of medication seemed to result in increased diarrhea, which eventually did not go away between infections. When Johnny was started on solids, he spat most of them out, and by the age of eighteen months, he would only accept yogurt with mashed banana, applesauce, small pieces of cheese toast, and scrambled eggs. His diarrhea continued and made it impossible for Jodie to take Johnny to any daytime classes such as swimming or gymnastics. Her frequent trips to her doctor did not produce any answers. At twenty-two months, Johnny developed yet another cold that resulted in his first asthma attack. He was taken to hospital by ambulance because his breathing was labored, but he recovered quickly when he was given the appropriate medication. Johnny was discharged with a diagnosis of asthma and placed on a number of medications, including a daily steroid inhaler to control his symptoms.

Jodie is now at her wit's end and completely exhausted from caring for Johnny. She has been forced to leave her job because she is not able to find anyone who can adequately meet all of Johnny's needs. The asthma diagnosis presented an additional challenge, and Jodie is reluctant to leave him with anyone but her husband.

The health of Jodie's baby and the stress level of her family would be dramatically improved if Johnny's food sensitivities were addressed. The trigger food is likely the dairy based foods consumed both by his mother when he was nursing and then eaten by him as he grew up. Soya appears to also be a potential problem which is common in dairy intolerant people, and Johnny would benefit from having only limited amounts of this food, as well. His symptoms will continue to worsen as he grows, and the impact on both his life and his family will be profound if his diet is not changed.

Julian, age seven: learning disabilities, ADHD, aggressive behavior, poor coordination, recurrent tonsillitis, and a chronically runny nose.

Julian has been a busy boy for as long as his parents, Heather and Lawrence, can remember. As a toddler, his attention span was so

3

short that he rarely stayed at any activity for more than a minute or two. Their house was always strewn with toys, and Julian insisted on climbing on everything. He suffered from bouts of tonsillitis almost every couple of months and his nose seemed to be perpetually running, even when he didn't seem to have a cold. He refused almost all the foods his parents offered with the exception of chicken nuggets, chicken noodle soup, and apple juice.

When he entered preschool, the kids were afraid of him on the playground, and he was quickly labeled as a bully. His aggressive behavior and refusal to wait his turn in the classroom resulted in him being isolated, and he rarely got invited to any birthday parties. Julian seemed accident-prone and was constantly falling and hurting himself. Both his fine motor and gross motor skills seemed delayed, and Heather and Lawrence were concerned about his readiness to attend kindergarten at the age of five. In addition, he continues to be sick often with tonsillitis and has been taking a least one course of antibiotics every three months since he was three. Heather is convinced that his behavior deteriorates after every course of antibiotics he has.

Julian is now in grade two and already showing signs of being academically and physically delayed. His fine motor skills are poor so he has difficulty holding his pencil and is usually slow getting his work done. During gym, the teacher comments that Julian is often uncooperative and inattentive. He has great difficulty doing exercises such as jumping jacks and often mixes up his left and right hand. In the classroom, Julian also finds it difficult to focus and often misunderstands the directions the teacher gives. Julian's parents are very concerned about his future.

Julian's story portrays the emotional and social impact of unaddressed food sensitivities. As he grows, these challenges will increase and his lack of academic and social success at school will put him at significant risk during his teenage years. By removing chicken which is the problem trigger food for Julian, both his behavioral and physical symptoms will improve. His self esteem will rise and he will no longer be viewed as a difficult child by his friends and his teachers.

Jennifer, age sixteen: acne, chronic bladder and yeast infections, migraines, irregular periods, and a very moody disposition.

Jennifer hates school. She hates sports. She hates doing chores. She actually dislikes most things except hanging out with her friends and listening to music on her iPhone. Her parents wonder what has happened to their little girl who used to have a sunny disposition and a sense of adventure. As a toddler, she had chronic bladder infections and recurrent tummy aches, but antibiotics seemed to keep things under control. She was also a very picky eater and refused almost everything her parents offered with the exception of crackers, toast, and cereal but she still seemed to be happy.

When Jennifer reached the age of twelve, however, it was as though someone had flipped a switch. All of a sudden her sunny disposition vanished and she became moody and argumentative, and her school performance deteriorated. She often skipped class and seemed to simply not care about the impact it was having on her marks. She developed severe acne and was placed on a long-term dose of antibiotics along with birth control pills, but these resulted in only minimal improvement. She began to have chronic yeast infections that required almost continuous medication and her periods were very erratic and unpredictable.

Now, at the age of fourteen, Jennifer's diet consists primarily of junk food, such as pizza, donuts, cakes and cookies, and she regularly gets severe migraine headaches. These headaches seem to be more common on the weekend after she has been out with her friends and are impacting her ability to spend time with her boyfriend. Jennifer's parents have been unable to find anyone who can offer an explanation why their daughter's health is deteriorating so significantly. Jennifer's attitude change and her decreasing interest in school are a source of worry for her parents as they are concerned about how this will impact her future.

Jennifer's story demonstrates how food sensitivities are impacted by the normal developmental changes that children go through. The hormonal changes that Jennifer experienced at puberty increased the impact of the foods that were already causing some other symptoms when she was younger. Removal of the gluten based products from her diet would result in significant improvement in both Jennifer's physical symptoms and her belligerent and argumentative attitude. Because of her age, it will be essential that her parents help Jennifer to find a strong and motivating reason to change her diet in order to enlist her cooperation. Because her symptoms are impacting her social life, Jennifer may be willing to cooperate. If the trigger food is not removed from Jennifer's diet, her challenging behavior and symptoms will continue into adulthood, and her future will be severely impacted.

FOOD SENSITIVITY SIGNS AND SYMPTOM CHECKLIST

One of the most effective tools in this book is the food sensitivity signs and symptoms checklist I have developed that you will find on the following pages. It is a common experience for clients of all ages to burst into tears when they see—often for the first time—a connection and common thread among the wide range of symptoms they have been experiencing. Many of the symptoms on this list will be ones that are not commonly associated with food. For example, while you may decide to try the diet because your child has chronic tummy aches, you may also find relief for his bedwetting, his crabby disposition, and his difficulty learning to read.

You will likely see your child as well as other members of your family reflected on this list. You may find yourself ticking boxes in almost every section, or you may notice that you have ticked a number of boxes that relate to one particular body system. Either way, this is indicative of a food sensitivity, and taking further steps to identify the trigger food and remove it from your child's diet will likely produce a dramatic improvement in their symptoms.

On the following pages is a list of many of the symptoms that can be related to food sensitivities. Along with the complete medical and family history and diet evaluation questionnaire found in chapter three, it is possible to identify an offending food that may be responsible for some of these problems. Removal of this food can often result in dramatic improvement in many of these symptoms. Mark the symptoms that are bothering your child now with a check mark, the ones that may have been a problem in the past with an X, and place the letter F beside symptoms that occur in you, your spouse, or other members of your child's extended family.

A. Skin

_____itching—any body part

_____eczema

_____recurrent hives

_____fungal infections (athlete's foot or genital infections)

_____excessive sweating, particularly at night

_____acne

_____family history of skin problems

_____skin rashes as a baby

_____recurrent red or flushed cheeks

_____dislike of being cuddled and touched

_____bright red buttocks as a baby or young child

_____small pimples on buttocks

_____scalded, red appearance on buttocks as a baby

_____brittle nails

_____hair loss

_____rapid development of hives following exposure to a food or other substance

B. Nervous System and Behavior

_____depression

_____headaches

_____migraines

_____difficulty sleeping

_____excessive tiredness

_____sensitivity to cold or heat

_____nightmares

_____mood swings

_____negative, apathetic attitude

_____difficulty learning sequential concepts, such as telling time

_____poor memory

_____difficulty remembering directions, particularly if they involve several steps

_____weak organizational skills

_____unexplained crying spells

_____angry outbursts

_____restlessness

_____short attention span

_____unusual twitches or tics

_____diagnosis of Tourette's syndrome

_____outbursts of foul language

_____unusual repetitive behaviors such as cracking knuckles, blinking eyes

_____learning disabilities

_____hyperactive behavior

_____born prematurely

_____excessive sensitivity to being touched

_____diagnosed with autism by a physician

_____restless legs

_____accident-prone

_____leads with the same foot when climbing stairs rather than alternating feet

_____stumbles and trips often and seems uncoordinated

_____excessively clingy as a child

_____craves a particular food excessively

_____anxiety

_____daytime sleepiness

_____desire to crouch or hide in small corners or under furniture

_____noticeable decrease in writing or reading ability after exposure to problem food or chemical

_____family history of alcoholism

_____delayed speech

_____reluctance to keep clothing on as a child

_____extremely active in utero before delivery

_____hyperactive behavior as an infant such as shaking crib, banging head, refusing to be held

_____as an infant, needed to be constantly walked or bounced in order to sleep

_____excessive tantrums

_____very easily frustrated by small events

C. Eyes and Vision

_____increased sensitivity to light

_____excessive blinking

_____excessive rubbing of eyes

_____tired, watery eyes

_____itchy or red eyes

_____dark circles under eyes

_____bags under eyes

_____wrinkles under the eye

_____difficulty following moving objects with both eyes at the same time

_____difficulty keeping place when reading

_____crossed eyes

_____"spaced out" look and appearance of being disconnected from their environment

D. Ears

_____chronic ear infections
_____decreased ability to hear
_____increased sensitivity to noise
_____ringing in the ears
_____repeated courses of antibiotics for ear infections
_____redness on the outside of one or both ears

E. Nose

_____chronic stuffy nose
_____chronic runny nose
_____repeated rubbing and itching of nose
_____excessive sneezing
_____repeated sinus infections
_____reduced or heightened sense of smell
_____recurrent nosebleeds
_____pain from blocked sinuses
_____hay fever
_____repeated use of antihistamines

F. Mouth and Throat

_____bad taste in mouth
_____bad breath
_____chronic tonsillitis
_____hoarse voice
_____persistent and recurrent canker sores
_____constant clearing of throat
_____swollen, red, cracked lips
_____excessive thirst, particularly for carbonated drinks
_____sucking on fingers or clothes
_____recurrent cold sores
_____thick, white coating on tongue or inside of cheeks

_____relentless talking and rambling on without a great deal of meaning

_____stuttering

_____excessive drooling as an infant

_____unusual moans, groans, or strange sounds repeated often

_____history of mouth infections, such as thrush

_____history of recurrent dental disease

_____feeling of having a lump in the throat

_____diagnosed with enlarged thyroid or underactive thyroid

G. Lungs

_____persistent cough during the day

_____persistent cough at night

_____family history of asthma

_____asthma (diagnosed by a doctor)

_____croup as a child

_____recurrent bronchitis

_____recurrent pneumonia

_____taking asthma medications

_____wheezing when exercising

_____wheezing in cold weather

_____shortness of breath when exercising or climbing stairs

_____rapid onset of respiratory distress symptoms upon contact with specific food or other substance

H. Digestive Tract

_____bloating and excessive gas

_____recurrent hiccoughs

_____increased or decreased appetite

_____itchy, red area around anus

_____recurrent diarrhea

_____recurrent constipation

_____chronic stomach aches

_____tendency to become overweight easily

_____underweight for age

_____soiling of underwear with stool

_____haemorrhoids

_____history of colic as an infant

_____family history of digestive complaints

_____chronic heartburn

_____repeated choking

_____history of low blood sugar

_____history of excessive spitting up as an infant

_____repeated vomiting as an infant or child

_____recurrent hiccoughs while baby in uterus of mother

_____stomach ulcers

_____gall bladder disease or removal of gall bladder

_____anorexia

_____bulimia

_____family history of eating disorders

_____diagnosed with irritable bowel syndrome

_____diagnosed with Crohn's disease

_____diagnosed with ulcerative colitis

_____diagnosed with any other bowel disease

_____episode of severe travelers diarrhea

I. Muscles and Joints

_____swollen feet and legs

_____cold hands and feet

_____muscle cramps and spasms during the day

_____muscle cramps at night

_____growing pains as a child

_____muscle stiffness, particularly in the morning

_____sore, aching muscles

_____muscle weakness on exertion

_____numbness in fingers or toes

_____fibromyalgia

_____autoimmune disease, such as systemic lupus, or ankylosing spondylitis _____slouches often and falls over if pushed even slightly when sitting or standing

_____difficulty performing exercises that require bilateral coordination, such as jumping jacks

_____walking by seven to ten months

_____sore or stiff joints

_____arthritis

J. Urinary and Genital Tract

_____frequent need to urinate

_____bedwetting past age three

_____wetting during the day past age three

_____urgent need to urinate

_____history of recurrent bladder infections

_____red, inflamed genital area

_____itchy genital area

_____heavy or irregular menstrual periods

_____increase or decrease in sex drive

_____genital sores

_____recurrent vaginal yeast infections

_____excessive pulling or rubbing of their genitals in infants or children

_____diagnosed with diabetes at age _____

_____family history of diabetes

_____prostate problems in men of extended family

_____abnormal menstruation

_____HIV-positive—child or other family members

_____infertility in child or other family members

K. Cardiovascular System

_____high blood pressure

_____high blood pressure in extended family member

_____higher than normal blood pressure as a child

_____rapid pulse

_____abnormally slow pulse without strong physical fitness
_____bruises easily
_____taking heart or blood pressure medication
_____irregular heartbeat
_____fluid retention
_____congenital heart disease in child
_____congenital heart disease in family member

Once you have completed this checklist, you should be able to determine if there is a good possibility that your child's health, behavior, or learning symptoms may be related to a food he or she is consuming. If you have checked off a number of symptoms, the chances are very high that your child would benefit from the identification of the trigger food along with removal of this food from his or her diet. Please continue reading the book, and take time to complete the extensive medical and family history form found in chapter three. Following completion of this form, you should be able to identify the hidden trigger food in your child's diet that is responsible for his or her symptoms. The remaining chapters of the book will offer step-by-step support in how to successfully remove this food in the midst of your already busy life. I encourage you to take the time to complete this process, as the benefits for your child and your family may be life-changing.

This checklist is not intended to suggest that all of these symptoms can be completely eliminated by a change in diet. It is still essential that you seek the help of a qualified medical practitioner and fully investigate the cause of your symptoms.

CHAPTER 1 HIGHLIGHTS

CLIENT STORIES

- Three stories to demonstrate the potential impact that food sensitivities can have on health, learning, and behaviour of children

FOOD SENSITIVITY SIGNS AND SYMPTOM CHECKLIST

- Reactions to food can occur in any system of the body
- Some people notice that their symptoms are grouped primarily within one body system while others notice that they have one or two symptoms affecting a wide range of body parts.
- There is a strong correlation between symptoms in your child and those in other members of your extended family, so it is important to identify both.
- Addressing the symptoms identified in this checklist by adjusting your child's diet may result in significant improvement. This process is not meant, however, to replace the care of a qualified medical professional or to suggest that all the diseases on this list will be completely relieved by diet change.
- Once this list has been completed, move on to chapter three which contains the medical and family history form in order to identify the offending trigger food.

CHAPTER TWO

HOW DID THIS HAPPEN TO MY FAMILY?

"All Diseases Begin in the Gut" (Hippocrates, 460–370 BC)

THE NORMAL DIGESTIVE TRACT

"The digestive system is like the roots of a tree. When the roots are diseased, the whole tree is affected. Nutrition, digestion, absorption, bacterial balance, and intestinal permeability all play interdependent functions in the health of the gastrointestinal tract and the health of the whole body" [2.]

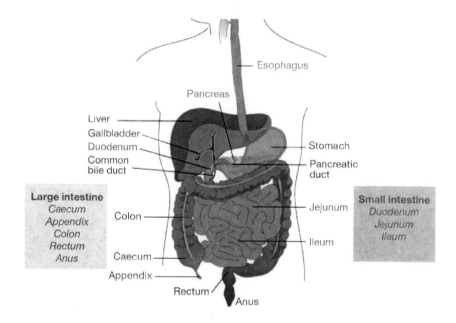

As you can see in the above diagram, the digestive tract (also known as the gastrointestinal tract) contains several organs as well as many complex muscles and glands. The job of the digestive tract is to break down the food we consume into a form from which the body can derive the energy and the nutrients that it needs.

The digestive tract contains 100 trillion bacteria, fungi, and microbes that are essential parts of digestion. It is the balance of all the parts of the digestive system working together that supports good health.[3] Anything that affects one part of the digestive tract has an impact on the functioning of the entire system and on the health of the entire body.

The Function of a Normal Digestive Tract

The digestive tract contains a number of organs that work together to digest the food that we eat, absorb the nutrients we need, and eliminate the waste products produced. It is a system that works very hard and processes 23,000 pounds of food over our lifetime.[4] The digestive system contains the following organs: mouth, esophagus, small and large intestines, gall bladder, liver, pancreas, rectum and anus.

Mouth

The food we eat begins by being chewed in the mouth and mixed with the salivary enzymes and mucous that is present there. These salivary glands produce approximately one litre of saliva per day which contains amylase, the enzyme that begins the digestion of the carbohydrates such as breads and fruits in our diet.[5] The mouth is also the body's first line of defense as it fights against bacteria and other organisms that enter our body from the outside.

Esophagus

From the mouth, the food then passes into the long, muscular tube called the esophagus. This tube pushes the food toward to the stomach by muscular contractions called peristalsis. The esophagus has a protective lining of cells that secrete mucous that offers lubrication and makes it easier for the food to pass in a downward direction. A valve at the bottom of the esophagus remains closed when food is not entering the stomach in order to prevent the acidic contents of the stomach from refluxing back into the esophagus and damaging the walls. This valve opens when food is passing through or when vomiting occurs.

Stomach

Once the food has passed through a valve called the cardiac sphincter at the base of the esophagus, it enters the stomach, which is located just below the diaphragm. The mucous membranes lining the stomach secrete a number of digestive juices and hydrochloric acid that help break down the ingested food and the muscular walls produce a churning action that helps break the food up into smaller pieces. It is here that a number of enzymes are secreted that aid in the digestion of protein and fat. The stomach lining also produces mucous, which offers a protective coating to the walls of the stomach from the acid contents it contains. Because the stomach can be exposed to organisms and harmful substances from the outside, the acid environment of the stomach also offers protection against these invaders by killing them.[6]

Small Intestine

The food then moves through a valve called the pyloric sphincter at the bottom of the stomach and into the small intestine, where more digestive juices are produced. The small intestine begins absorption of the nutrients and the water that the body needs for energy and cell growth, and these substances then pass into the bloodstream through the bowel wall.

This part of the intestine is over twenty feet in length and is divided into three distinct sections—the duodenum, the jejunum, and the ileum. Each of these sections has a unique function in the process of digestion. Most of the chemical digestion of our food occurs in the first section, known as the duodenum, as this is where the pancreas empties its digestive juice and where the liver empties bile for the digestion of fats.[7]

The mucous lining of the small intestine is made up of thousands and thousands of small folds that increase the surface area for absorption. These folds are covered with many small, finger-like protrusions called villi. Each of these small villi contain blood vessels that absorb the products of both carbohydrate and protein digestion. Each villi is also covered by a brush-like border that further increases absorption of the nutrients our body needs. These villi can be damaged in inflammatory bowel disease, when the balance of bowel bacteria is altered and also in response to the ingestion of poorly tolerated foods. When this damage occurs, the bowel is unable to digest and absorb food properly which leads to malabsorption, nutritional deficiencies, and food intolerances.[7] The cells of the small bowel also have the ability to produce a thick coating of mucous to protect this sensitive lining if substances causing irritation are present. This poses an additional problem because this mucous lining covers over the villi and thus prevents the absorption of nutrients and the breakdown of carbohydrates.

The mucous linings of the small and large bowel also serve another essential function. In healthy individuals, the epithelial cells that line the digestive tract are close together and are designed to allow only substances of a certain size to be absorbed into the bloodstream. Harmful by-products and undigested food are prevented from being absorbed and remain in the digestive tract to be excreted out of the body. If the bowel is inflamed, the space between these epithelial cells increases and particles of a much greater size are allowed to leak into the bloodstream and then circulate around the body before they are completely digested. This can result in the appearance of symptoms in any part of the body, and this is the process that occurs in food intolerances. It is commonly known as "leaky gut".

Because the small intestine is also exposed to food from the outside environment, it contains special cells that are capable of killing the bacteria and other organisms that were not dealt with in the stomach. Substances such as fibre plus other waste products that are not completely digested move into the large intestine by muscular contractions called peristalsis.

Large Intestine Including Rectum and Anus

The large intestine is only about five feet in length but has a much wider diameter than the small intestine. Undigested and unabsorbed food material enters the first section of the large intestine, known as the caecum, by passing through a sphincter known as the ileocecal valve. The appendix, which is a small pouch that is attached to the caecum, serves no function in digestion but is believed to be part of the immune system. Following the caecum, the other parts of the large intestine are the colon, the rectum, and the anus. Because some of the water and many of the nutrients and salts were removed in the small intestine, the consistency of the material as it enters the large intestine is slightly more solid.[8.]

The contents of the large intestine are acted upon by the large number of bacteria it contains, and these have a number of important functions. They help further break down the remaining material that was not completely broken down earlier in digestion, and they are responsible for the synthesis of Vitamin K and some B Vitamins, as well.[9] These vitamins are essential for good health and are absorbed from the large intestine into the bloodstream to be used by the body. The bacteria in the large intestine are meant to be present in a very specific balance. This balance is essential for them to be able to assist in the process of digestion and to help prevent the overgrowth of other disease-causing organisms. If this balance is disturbed because of inflammation, an unhealthy diet, consumption of antibiotics, or chronic stress, bad bacteria and yeast are permitted to overgrow. The toxic by-products from these organisms further tax the body and compromise digestion and are a major reason for the symptoms of food sensitivity.

The fungus Candida is the most common one to overgrow when the balance in the bowel is disturbed, and it is responsible for many systemic symptoms. The roots from this organism actually puncture the lining of the intestine as well as secrete acids that change the acid/base balance in the body and result in leaky gut.[10] It is important to take steps to improve digestion and restore the balance of the bacteria in the large bowel in order to treat food sensitivities. Taking probiotics containing good bacteria such as Lactobacillus and Bifidobacteria is one of the ways to achieve this.

The large intestine does not contain any folds of villi like the small intestine, so the surface area available for absorption is limited. By the time the remaining waste products reach the end of the large intestine, they should be quite solid in nature, and are stored in the rectum until they are then released from the body through the anus. This process may take three to five days.

Pancreas

The pancreas is a small organ that has an essential job in the digestion of our food and in the regulation of some of the hormones in our body. It produces pancreatic juice that contains enzymes that digest proteins, fats, and carbohydrates as well as bicarbonate that neutralizes the hydrochloric acid that enters the small intestine from the stomach. The secretions of the pancreas are emptied into the digestive system into the first section of the small intestine, called the duodenum.[11.]

The pancreas also contains specific cells called the Islets of Langerhans that secrete hormones directly into the bloodstream that are required to regulate blood sugar. Insulin is secreted to lower the blood sugar, and glucagon is secreted to elevate it.

Liver and Gallbladder

The liver is the largest gland in the body and creates bile that is used to digest the fats in our diet. When food containing fat is not being eaten, the bile produced by the liver is concentrated and stored in the gall bladder. When fat enters the small intestine, it initiates a mechanism that contracts the gallbladder and forces the bile into the small intestine. It is common for people to develop small stones that block this duct leading from the gall bladder to the small intestine, and this can produce severe pain, nausea, and vomiting. Bile is also an alkaline substance that helps to neutralize the stomach acid that enters the small intestine.

The liver also synthesizes several kinds of proteins and then releases them back into the blood. Two of these proteins, called prothrombin and fibrinogen, are important in the clotting of our blood. It is also the primary place in our body where detoxification takes place. All the blood of the body passes through the liver, and it removes harmful substances of all kinds. Substances such as hormones and environmental chemicals are meant to be deactivated in the liver and removed from the body, but if the liver is not functioning adequately, a buildup of chemicals, toxins, and hormones may result in a wide variety of symptoms.[12.]

THE IMMUNE SYSTEM AND THE DIGESTIVE TRACT

The body contains many specialized cells that allow it to absorb nutrients from the food that we eat without responding to it as a foreign substance. This GALT tissue (gut-associated lymphoid tissue) present throughout the bowel walls allows the body to differentiate between healthy, nutrient dense food and disease causing organisms. This lymphoid tissue is called Peyer's patches and is present in the small intestine and other types of lymph tissue in the appendix, the large intestine, the liver, and the esophagus. This system moves fluids, bacteria, and other harmful materials from the cells to lymph nodes throughout the body to be destroyed and eliminated.[13.]

If, however, the walls of the bowel become inflamed or the bacteria balance is disturbed, a wide variety of symptoms throughout the body may result. Because seventy percent of the immune system of your body is actually contained in your bowel, anything that causes inflammation in your digestive tract can potentially result in a decrease in your body's ability to fight off disease.[14] "On the whole it is hard to overestimate how important the state of our gut flora in the appropriate functioning of our immune system. The gut wall with its bacterial layer can be described as the right hand of the immune system. If the bacterial layer is damaged, or, worse than that, abnormal, then the person's immune system is trying to function with its right hand tied behind its back."[15.]

THE MIND-BODY-BOWEL CONNECTION

The function of the digestive system is controlled by a complex hormone system. These hormones are released, however, as a result of stimulation by the nervous system. One half of the nerves of the body are located in the digestive tract, and there is a direct connection through the vagus nerve from the brain down the entire length of the digestive tract. Even some of the neurotransmitters that determine our mood are produced in the digestive tract. "The digestive tract actually has about the same number of neurotransmitters as the brain, and we have more nerve cells in the bowel than in the spine"[16.]

Some of the nerves that control digestion are located outside the digestive system in the spinal cord and the brain, and some are contained within the bowel walls. Both of these sets of nerves determine the process and the speed with which food is processed throughout the body.

Because the bowel contains a "mind of its own," it is able to carry out its task without conscious thought on our part. Our bowels often respond to the stresses of our lives, and symptoms such as nausea and diarrhea are common warning signs that we are feeling pressured in some aspect of our lives. When stress becomes chronic, the symptoms often increase because our bodies are not physiologically adapted for ongoing, chronic stress. The fight-or-flight response that we experience when the threat of immediate danger occurs is intended to be short-lived, and our body cannot maintain the sense of alertness over extended periods of time.

During times of stress, our bodies mobilize their resources by increasing blood flow to our brains so we can think clearly, increasing our blood sugar so we have energy to run, increasing our heart rates and breathing rates so we have the power we need to fight, and by shutting down our digestive system, as it is not required as we flee from our enemies. The problem is that many of us live in states of chronic stress, and our bodies struggle to adapt for this prolonged period of time. Our bodies feel tired, our blood sugar plummets, our digestive systems complain, we struggle to think clearly, and we feel exhausted and unable to cope any longer. Our immune systems are also compromised, and we begin to experience the symptoms of any number of diseases.

When our health is severely compromised and our food has become a trigger for digestive disturbances, our brains can be affected in another way. When the balance of bacteria in our bowel is disturbed, the toxins produced by the over growth of bad bacteria can have a direct impact on our thought processes and our moods. These toxins are absorbed from the bowel into the blood stream and then reach our brain to produce symptoms. Poorly tolerated foods can also produce local inflammatory reactions that occur in the tissues of the brain and can be responsible for such symptoms as depression, anxiety, inability to sleep, nervous tics and behavior, and other neurological symptoms. Even stress, by itself, can result in the release of inflammatory chemicals in our bowels, such as histamine—even without contact with a poorly tolerated food—and produce a wide range of unpleasant symptoms.

"An unknown number of neurotoxins are produced by abnormal flora in the gut of children and adults, which get absorbed through the damaged gut wall into the blood and taken to the brain . . . these are the kinds of toxins which can make anybody mentally ill"[17]

This imbalance of bowel bacteria and decrease in the enzymes required for digestion also results in an additional concern for children and adults suffering from autism. The incomplete digestion of both dairy and gluten based foods produces by-products that are similar in structure to the opiate drugs such as morphine and heroin. These by-products are absorbed through the leaky bowel wall into the blood stream and eventually reach the brain. These substances have a dramatic impact on the nervous system and are responsible for the strong addiction these children often have to gluten and dairy based foods. The leaky gut that is common in children with autism is considered by many to be one of the major issues that needs to be addressed in order for these children to get well. More information on this topic is contained in chapter seven on autism.

PLACES WHERE DIGESTION CAN GO WRONG

Because so many essential nutrients and many of our hormone, neurotransmitter, and immune-building cells are contained in our digestive tract, disturbances in this system can have a significant impact on our health.

1. If the number of enzymes available to digest our food is decreased due to inflammation, the food progresses through the digestive tract without complete digestion and produces additional irritation in an already inflamed bowel.

2. If the balance of bacteria is upset and the bad bacteria proliferate at the expense of the good ones, digestion is again affected, and dangerous toxins produced by these organisms are absorbed into the body.

3. When foods are eaten that cause an adverse immune reaction or inflammation in the bowel, the bowel wall becomes inflamed, and the lining begins to leak. The breakdown products of food that would otherwise not be absorbed through the bowel wall into the bloodstream leak through and circulate through the body, causing a multitude of symptoms in a variety of other organs. This is known as leaky gut syndrome. Nutrition is compromised as the bacteria required to produce some of the vitamins are missing, and the nutrients from the foods that are eaten may not be adequately absorbed by the body.

WHY THINGS MIGHT GO WRONG IN THE DIGESTIVE TRACT

There are many things that impact the digestive tract and result in a wide variety of both digestive and other systemic symptoms.

1. Early consumption of cow's milk products and other foods before the digestive tract and the immune system of an infant have had time to mature to the point where they are tolerated

2. Doses of antibiotics, cortisone, birth control pills, or anti-inflammatory drugs that upset the natural balance of bacteria in the bowel and increase bowel wall inflammation

3. Stress that results in the alteration of the function of the digestive tract that then has a profound impact on other organs of the body

4. Serious illnesses or flu symptoms that cause severe diarrhea and result in damage to the lining of the bowel and a decrease in enzyme secretion

5. Advancing age, as enzyme production and peristalsis decrease with age

6. Consumption of foods a person is intolerant to that cause bowel inflammation and irritation, particularly if consumed on a repeated basis

7. Autoimmune disease that results in the body attacking the cells of its own digestive tract

8. A diet that is loaded with fat and highly processed food and deficient in fruits, vegetables, and fibre

9. A family history of diseases such as celiac disease that put the patient at risk for developing a bowel disease

10. Chronic constipation that results in toxins being retained in the bowel longer and causing increased inflammation

11. Exposure to toxic chemicals in the environment

DEFINITIONS OF FOOD SENSITIVITIES, ALLERGIES, AND INTOLERANCES

Food sensitivities are defined as any adverse reaction to food, no matter what the physiological mechanism involved. It is a general term that does not identify why the reaction is occurring or what types of symptoms result. There are two distinct and different types of reactions to food that make up this general category and it is important to understand the differences between them. These two types of reactions are known as food allergies and food intolerances.

Food Allergies[18.]

Many people use the term allergy to describe any adverse reaction they experience to either a food or another environmental substance. This term is often used incorrectly and confused with food intolerances which are the result of a local response to food in the bowel with no immune based reaction. An allergy occurs when the immune system of the body is mobilized in response to a foreign substance. This substance may be a food that is normally tolerated but, because of some malfunction in the body, a reaction is mobilized and symptoms result.

Because an understanding of the process involved in food allergies is essential in order to treat the symptoms that result, a brief summary is presented here. The important point to remember is that the antibody IgE is the one produced in true food allergies and the one that is measured in traditional skin and blood allergy tests.

1. A food or other substance enters the body and a determination is made about whether it is a foreign or safe substance.
2. If the substance is considered safe, no reaction results.
3. If the food or other substance is considered to be a threat, the body produces lymphocytes (a type of white blood cell) in response. These cells are the gatekeeper of the body's immune system.
4. There are two types of lymphocytes produced to assist the body to mobilize a reaction and eliminate the offender—T-cells and B-cells.
5. The T-cells are able to create two different types of response within the body, depending on the type of invader they must react to.
6. A T-1 response is mobilized in order for the body to successfully deal with a disease producing organism and destroy it. Antibodies known as IgG are produced by the B-cells in response.
7. A T-2 response is mobilized if the substance is recognized as an allergen such as a food and antibodies known as IgE are produced by the B-cells.
8. IgE antibodies are responsible for the release of histamine and other chemicals in allergic reactions and the inflammation that results.
9. Histamine is produced in the body by mast cells that are present in the digestive tract, lungs, skin and respiratory tract and released in response to IgE production.

10. As well as producing T-cells, the body also produces B-cells in response to a foreign substance. These B-cells produce the antibodies used throughout the body to respond to foreign substances of all kinds.
11. There are five types of antibodies produced—IgG, IgA, IgM, IgE, and IgD.
12. Traditional allergy testing focuses on the identification of foods producing an IgE response.
13. Some blood tests for food sensitivities focus on the identification of IgG antibodies but these tests remain controversial and the results are inconsistent and often inaccurate.

The foreign substance in an allergic reaction is known as an antigen, and a specific antibody is produced by the body to eliminate it. We have a large number of circulating antibodies in our body, waiting to connect to and neutralize the foreign substances that we continually come in contact with. They are like a lock and key where a specific antigen meets up with a specific antibody and attempts to destroy it. When an antigen and antibody combine, the result is the release of histamine and other chemicals which are the cause of the troubling symptoms present in allergic reactions. Because of this release of histamine, an antihistamine medication usually results in a dramatic improvement in the symptoms.

Characteristics of food allergies:

1. They occur in up to eight percent of children under the age of five. The incidence goes up when there is a family history of allergies.
2. It is believed that only two percent of adults have true allergies to foods.
3. The reaction is almost always immediate.
4. The reaction is usually consistent and predictable each time the person is exposed to the allergen.

5. The symptoms are more likely to be localized and acute rather than affecting multiple parts of the body initially. For example, a life-threatening response to peanuts initially appears as a tightening of the muscles of the throat, mouth, and airway.

6. Symptoms are not usually dose-related. Even a small amount of the offending food usually produces symptoms.

7. Once you have been exposed to a specific antigen, your body continues to have the corresponding antibody circulating so that it reacts quickly when exposed again.

8. The most common antibody in allergies is IgE, which is one of the five immunglobulins produced by the lymphocytes, one of the groups of the white blood cells.

9. Some of the blood and scratch tests specific for IgE are often able to identify foods causing an allergic reaction.

10. The symptoms of allergies are caused by the release of inflammatory chemicals such as histamine, which are destructive substances that attempt to destroy the invading antigen. These inflammatory chemicals react with the tissues of the body to produce inflammation.

11. Some symptoms can be life-threatening emergencies and require immediate medical attention. Epi—pens should be carried by all people who may experience these severe symptoms, and those who have allergies should be trained to use them at the first sign of a reaction.

12. Symptoms are often relieved by taking an antihistamine to counteract the histamine that has been released.

13. The most common foods that cause anaphylactic reactions in children are peanuts, shellfish, milk, and eggs. It is possible, however, for a child to experience an allergic reaction to any food, chemical or environmental substance.

14. Exercise may increase the reaction to a food and cause an allergic reaction, but the mechanism is not well understood.

Food Intolerances[19.]

Food intolerances are caused by a reaction to a food that does not result in the mobilization of an immune response. The list of steps produced in an allergic reaction does not occur. The symptoms are the result of any of a number of possible causes of disturbance in the functioning of the digestive tract such as the consumption of poorly tolerated or unhealthy foods, the balance of bacteria, inadequate enzyme production, or the overgrowth of Candida or another organism. Anything that causes inflammation and irritation results in what is known as leaky gut. When the bowel wall becomes leaky, substances are absorbed through the bowel wall without being completely digested and are recognized by the body as foreign substances. These substances enter the bloodstream and circulate throughout the body to create symptoms in a wide variety of organs. Unlike allergies, food intolerances are more difficult to diagnose, and it believed that at least 50 percent of people have intolerances to some foods. The symptoms caused by food intolerances have several characteristics that differentiate them from allergies, and this distinction is important in determining what treatment is undertaken. While the immune system of the body is not involved in the reaction to the food, the immune system is compromised when poorly tolerated foods are consumed. Because seventy per cent of the immune system is contained in the bowel, when these tissues become inflamed, the immune system is affected.

Characteristics of food intolerances:

1. The symptoms are the result of anything that causes local inflammation and irritation in the bowel but does not result in an immune response and release of the immunoglobulin IgE.
2. Traditional allergy tests that measure the level of specific IgE reactions to foods are not helpful in diagnosis, as no IgE is produced.
3. People may develop a specific food intolerance because of an enzyme deficiency, such as the enzyme lactase that

digests the sugar in milk. The breakdown of complex sugars is compromised when the bowel is inflamed. Digestive enzymes decrease with age and can produce severe diarrhea in elderly people in response to some foods, particularly dairy products.

4. Reactions can be delayed as much as twenty-four or even seventy-two hours.

5. The reaction is not always predictable, because it is also related to other aspects of the person's life. If someone is under chronic stress, eats more than one poorly tolerated food at once, has some type of other illness, or is taking any medications that affect the digestive tract, that person is more likely to develop symptoms.

6. Symptoms can be related to the quantity of the food that is eaten. Unlike allergies, a small amount of a food eaten infrequently may be tolerated even when larger quantities are not. There is usually a threshold of tolerance where symptoms appear.

7. Symptoms most often involve multiple body systems. It is not uncommon that, over time, as the body's ability to adapt decreases, acute symptoms decrease to be replaced by a chronic, nonspecific sense of fatigue and malaise in addition to other, more specific symptoms.

8. Symptoms are rarely life-threatening on the short term

9. Taking an antihistamine is of no value, because these reactions do not produce histamine.

10. The usual method of detection is through the use of a multiple food elimination diet. This diet has a very low compliance rate except in severe food allergies, and many foods are missed through this method. Because the response to food intolerance may be delayed for forty-eight hours or more, it is crucial that only one food be added back to the diet at a time with a number of days in between to ensure there has not been a reaction.

11. Some food intolerances can be the result of naturally occurring substances or food additives in foods. Some

people are intolerant to the naturally occurring histamine in foods, so they require diets that remove these foods. Because everyone has a threshold of tolerance for histamine, they can often tolerate small quantities of these foods if eaten one at a time. These responses are usually due to a deficiency in the enzyme that is needed to process the histamine, and tolerance for these foods can be increased if this enzyme is taken orally when these foods are eaten.

FACTORS CONTRIBUTING TO THE DEVELOPMENT OF FOOD SENSITIVITIES

There are many factors that determine the development of food sensitivities. Sometimes one individual factor is significant enough to result in symptoms, but more often, they are the result of a combination of factors working together. The history form that you will be completing in chapter three of this book includes extensive questions related to each of these specific topics. In order to accurately identify the trigger food that is creating the symptoms for your child or other members of your family, it is important to consider all the information contained in the history form together rather than make a quick judgment based on incomplete information.

1. **Family history:** A strong family history of symptoms suggestive of food-related issues is a common pattern in patients. It is often the case, however, that many family members have health and emotional concerns that have never been resolved nor had the cause identified. Particularly when looking back two generations or more, the complaints are often vague, but common family symptoms are still visible. In many situations, I have seen families with a long history of a particular disease where it is assumed that the disease is simply a common family trait. It is often discovered, however, that it is not the disease that is the common thread, but the sensitivity to a certain food. An example of this can be seen in families with a longstanding history of asthma and respiratory disorders. When I look closer

and ask a few more questions, it is actually clear that almost everyone has been intolerant to milk in some form and often over-consumes it in another. It is the intolerance to dairy products that is the family link and not the asthma or chronic bronchitis. An extensive family history is an essential part of identifying the trigger food.

2. **Effects on infants during pregnancy:** The diets and lifestyles of pregnant women are very important in determining the health of their newborn children. Poor nutrition and excessive stress have been well documented to impact the immune systems and the physical development of babies. In addition, foods consumed by the mother that she is sensitive to also have an impact on the unborn child. It is common to hear from mothers that their baby had recurrent hiccups while she was pregnant and that these continue when the child consumes cow's milk products after birth. Removal by the mother of foods that she is significantly intolerant to during her pregnancy dramatically decreases the chance of future intolerances by the child.

3. **Method of feeding:** The early introduction of cow's milk into the diet of many children can result in significant digestive disturbances. The infant's immune system and digestive tract are not able to tolerate foreign proteins at an early age, and many children develop colic, diarrhea, and chronic ear and chest infections as a result. Almost 50 percent of children who are bothered by cow's milk are also bothered by soya milk, so symptoms may persist despite a change to a soya-based formula. Breast milk is definitely the milk of choice for babies but the diet of the mother has an impact on the health and behavior of her infant. If a mother eats foods that she is sensitive to, the baby may experience digestive upsets and colic. Removal of offending foods as well as rotation of what the mother eats most often eliminates these symptoms. Mothers of colicky newborns are usually exhausted and feel inadequate in their new role as parents, so identifying the trigger food and supporting them to

remove this food from their diet makes a tremendous difference in their lives. As a mother of a baby who cried day and night for three months and slept no longer than twenty minutes at a time, I am committed to ensuring that all new mothers know that altering their diet can have a huge impact on their baby, the amount of sleep everyone gets, and the peace within their family.

4. **Introduction of solid food:** It is now common practice to delay the introduction of solid food until after an infant is six months old. This allows the digestive system to mature to the point where it is able to tolerate a wider range of foods. The cells in the bowel wall are then snugly closed and no longer allow undigested particles of food to be absorbed into the body. This also allows time for the digestive enzymes required to develop. It is important to follow the recommended sequence of introducing foods with the avoidance of the common offenders such as eggs, peanuts, citrus fruits, shellfish, dairy products, and wheat until the child is at least a year old. New foods introduced too early or too many at a time may result in digestive complaints and other health concerns in the baby. In addition, parents should avoid giving their child, during their first year of their life, any food that others in their family are bothered by. The chances of the child also being bothered by this food are higher than normal, and the child would benefit from this food being introduced only when they are older. The parents can simply substitute a healthy, age appropriate alternative in its place.

5. **Current diet and nutritional status:** It is essential for our body to receive the nutrients it needs for growth and for repair of tissues. If the diet consumed is deficient in many vitamins and minerals and does not contain adequate fibre, the function of the bowel is affected, and absorption of nutrients from the food we eat is decreased. As digestion is impacted, some of the foods we eat create inflammation, and a wide variety of symptoms may result. Many children with food sensitivities are

very picky eaters and eat only a very select number of foods. This is an important clue, because the food that is causing their symptoms is usually the one they crave and the one they over-consume. As they repeatedly eat this food, the walls of their bowels become inflamed and irritated, and a number of symptoms usually appear. Once the poorly tolerated food is removed from their diets, their bodies begin to heal, and they are willing to try a wider range of food. There is often a dramatic change in the variety of the diet of the child, and their overall health improves, because they are obtaining more balanced nutrition.

6. **Multiple doses of antibiotics:** While antibiotics are very effective in killing bacteria that cause serious infections, they also have a major impact on the balance of good bacteria in the bowel. Multiple infections resulting in multiple antibiotics can have a very serious impact of the health of the digestive tract. If children are having multiple ear or chest infections requiring antibiotics, it is important to investigate the possibility that they have a sensitivity to something they are eating that is the underlying cause of their problem. Many doctors prescribe antibiotics unnecessarily for viral illnesses in children. It is important to be sure your child has a bacterial infection that will benefit from the antibiotics rather than a simple viral infection that will go away on its own.

7. **Autoimmune diseases and diseases of the digestive tract:** There are many diseases that result in damage and inflammation in the digestive tract. Even diarrhea caused by a bad case of the flu can result in either short-term or long-term intolerances to certain foods. During a bout of serious diarrhea, it is essential to avoid dairy products, as the enzyme lactase that digests the sugar lactose in milk is usually destroyed. Consumption of dairy products often results in a worsening of the symptom. It is preferable to have clear soups and juices or flat pop such as 7UP or ginger ale. In breastfed babies with serious diarrhea, it

may even be necessary for the mother to express her milk and add lactose-digesting drops to her milk before she feeds it back to her baby.

There are many other diseases of the digestive tract that can be both the cause and result of food sensitivities. The severe diarrhea of diseases such as Crohn's disease, ulcerative colitis, and irritable bowel syndrome increases the chance of food sensitivities as they damage the bowel wall.[20.] There is also evidence now that many digestive and autoimmune diseases can be dramatically improved if trigger foods are removed from the diet. Considering the severity of these diseases, giving diet manipulation a try is worthwhile.

In my own personal experience, the autoimmune disease that I have as a result of a severe E.coli infection I had over twenty years ago is dramatically improved when I avoid grains and dairy products. Many of my clients with digestive and autoimmune diseases have experienced a dramatic improvement in their symptoms when trigger foods were removed from their diet.

8. **Medications:** There are many medications that cause irritation and inflammation in the bowel. Common over-the-counter medications such as Ibuprofen can result in an upset stomach and even ulcers if they are not taken with food. In addition, many chronic illnesses require large doses of medications that have a significant impact on the bowel, and patients need to receive careful instructions on how and when to take these pills. It is often common for patients to develop digestive symptoms that are attributed to their disease when the symptoms are due to the side effects of the pills or to a food intolerance.

9. **Life Stresses:** The bowel is very sensitive to our emotional state. Chronic stress results in a fight-or-flight response and puts our bodies in a constant state of alertness. When this happens, our digestive systems shut down, because in the days of the

caveman, we did not require digestion as we escaped from the woolly mammoth. Chronic stress results in incomplete digestion of food that is eaten and a multitude of digestive complaints. While removal of trigger foods from a diet can result in significant improvement, unless the severe stress in the person's life is attended to, the improvement is often short-lived, as other offending foods begin to reappear. This topic is addressed in later sections of the book, and tools are offered both to assess the level of your stress and to find healthier strategies for coping.

Real-Life Story

The following story illustrates the multitude of symptoms and parts of the body that can be affected by food sensitivities. The social and emotional results of these symptoms often have a huge impact on the lives of both adults and children. This story demonstrates clearly the long term implications for adults when food sensitivities are not addressed in their childhood.

Mary Jane is a sixty-year-old mother of three adult children and three young grandchildren. She has worked hard throughout her life and is now hoping to enjoy her recent retirement. Unfortunately her health has deteriorated to the point where she barely drags herself through her day. She has recently been diagnosed with fibromyalgia after years of overwhelming fatigue, sore joints, and migraine headaches.

As she reflects back over her life, she can hardly remember a time when she felt 100 percent well. Even as a child, she suffered from eczema, stomach aches and exercise-induced asthma and seemed to be forever seeing one doctor or another. She took huge doses of antibiotics for her acne as a teenager and was even put on the birth control pill at the age of fourteen in an effort to improve the severe PMS from which she suffered. By the time she graduated from high school, she had gained twenty-five extra pounds, and her self-confidence was severely lacking. She tried to attend university but found that her ability to remember what she was learning was poor, so she finally quit in frustration.

When Mary Jane married and again went back on the birth control pill, she was plagued by vaginal yeast infections, and her digestive tract seemed to protest against everything she ate. She stopped the pill and went on to have three children over the next five years. All of her children were colicky babies who were often ill with multiple ear infections, chronic diarrhea, and behavior challenges. Mary Jane's mother commented to her that it was like living her own infancy over again. It seems that Mary Jane had also been a colicky baby with ear infections requiring antibiotics herself.

Mary Jane is now hoping her life and the lives of her family members will be transformed by addressing their individual food sensitivities. In the book she found yesterday at the bookstore, she discovered stories very similar to her own. The author has developed a process of identifying trigger foods that may be responsible for the many chronic symptoms that have been having such a negative impact on Mary Jane's life.

CHAPTER 2 HIGHLIGHTS

THE NORMAL DIGESTIVE TRACT

- The digestive system is like the roots of a tree. If the roots are diseased, the entire tree is affected.
- Nutrition, digestion, absorption, bacterial balance, and intestinal permeability all play interdependent functions in the health of the gastrointestinal tract and the health of the whole body.
- The digestive system contains the following organs: mouth, esophagus, small and large intestines, gall bladder, liver, pancreas, rectum and anus.
- The digestive tract contains 100 trillion bacteria, fungi, and microbes that are essential parts of digestion.
- The job of the digestive tract is to break down the food we consume into a form from which the body can derive the energy and nutrients it needs.

THE IMMUNE SYSTEM AND THE DIGESTIVE TRACT

- Seventy percent of the immune system of your body is actually contained in your bowel, so anything that causes inflammation in your digestive tract can potentially result in a decrease in your body's ability to fight off disease.

THE MIND-BODY-BOWEL CONNECTION

- One half of the nerves of the body are located in the digestive tract.
- The digestive tract actually has about the same number of neurotransmitters as the brain, and we have more nerve cells in the bowel than in the spine.
- Because the bowel contains a "mind of its own," it is able to carry out its task without conscious thought on our part.

- Food sensitivities can also produce inflammatory reactions that occur in the tissues of the brain and can be responsible for such symptoms as depression, anxiety, inability to sleep, nervous tics, and behavior and other neurological symptoms.
- Stress, by itself, can result in the release of inflammatory chemicals in our bowels, such as histamine—even without contact with a poorly tolerated food—and result in a wide range of unpleasant symptoms.

PLACES WHERE DIGESTION CAN GO WRONG

- Because so many essential nutrients and many of our hormone, neurotransmitter, and immune-building cells are contained in our digestive tracts, disturbances in this system can have a significant impact on our health.

WHY THINGS MIGHT GO WRONG
IN THE DIGESTIVE TRACT

- Early consumption in infancy of foods poorly tolerated
- Multiple doses of antibiotics, anti-inflammatory drugs, steroids, or other medications and substances that upset the balance of bacteria or irritate the lining of the digestive tract
- Stress
- Prolonged diarrhea or chronic constipation
- Advancing age
- Consumption of poorly tolerated foods
- Autoimmune diseases such as rheumatoid arthritis, systemic lupus, or Crohn's disease

DEFINITIONS OF FOOD SENSITIVITIES, ALLERGIES, AND INTOLERANCES

- Food sensitivities occur when someone reacts adversely to a food, no matter whether the mechanism is an allergy or an intolerance.
- Food allergies are a response to a food where the immune system is involved.
- Food allergies occur in about eight percent of children under five and two percent of adults.
- Food allergies can be identified through traditional skin and blood tests.
- Food intolerance is a response to a food by the body when the immune system is not the cause of the reaction.
- Food intolerances are responsible for most of the reactions people experience to foods that they eat.
- There are no accurate tests to determine food intolerances except a trial removal of the offending food.

FACTORS CONTRIBUTING TO THE DEVELOPMENT OF FOOD SENSITIVITIES

- Family history
- Impact on the infant during pregnancy
- Method of feeding
- Time of introduction of solid food and the type of food introduced
- Current diet and nutritional status
- Multiple doses of antibiotics
- Autoimmune diseases and diseases of the digestive tract
- Medications
- Life stresses

CHAPTER THREE

HOW DO I KNOW WHAT FOOD TO REMOVE?

I often see families who have been trying desperately to uncover hidden food sensitivities and have found the entire experience exhausting and frustrating. They read a book or an article or hear from a friend or professional that food might be part of the cause of their child's health, learning, or behavior challenges, but they find it almost impossible to navigate the path to figure out what food it might be. I see many clients who have been placed on elimination diets but simply couldn't figure out how to remove the ten or more foods suggested by the doctor. Their families refused to eat the lamb, blueberries, and rice they were allowed at the start of the elimination diet, and school lunches were impossible to make with all the restrictions. It is a common story to hear that they removed eight of the ten foods that were on the list given to them by the doctor, but despite their valiant efforts, their children are no better. They often abandon the entire process and never return for their follow-up appointments or return and simply lie and say it didn't work.

45

I have also seen many clients who have undertaken unpleasant allergy testing with their children only to learn, as I did, that most foods are not true allergies and aren't picked up by that type of testing. Most symptoms related to food do not involve the release of histamine by the body when they are eaten, so the standard allergy tests that measure the amount of histamine released are of little diagnostic value. Most food reactions are called intolerances and are caused by local inflammation in the bowel rather than by the immune system. There is a complete explanation of this process in chapter two of this book. Many parents follow the well-meaning advice of a professional who insists their child isn't bothered by milk if the allergy skin test is negative, even if the child experiences symptoms each time he or she eats it. Some physicians have the attitude that it is impossible to feed a child a nutritious diet without common foods such as milk or wheat, so they discourage parents from even giving it a try.

THE TRIGGER FOOD CONCEPT

As I have worked hard to understand the food sensitivities of both my own family members and countless clients, I have designed a process of identifying the trigger food that is exceptionally accurate. While I support everyone seeking the help of medical professionals to ensure that their child is thoroughly investigated for any serious illnesses, I believe that searching for food sensitivities has to be manageable within the context of the real life of parents and their children. I have watched hundreds of families give up after only a few days of attempting to identify the foods that were bothering their children as they found it overwhelming. I have spent many years exploring alternative ways of identifying offending foods. This book follows the process that I have designed and used over the last twenty-five years, and I am very successful in uncovering the hidden trigger food. This approach also helps children get well while eating a healthy and balanced diet, as it removes only one or two foods and is manageable in the lives of families.

The concept is simple: rather than search for or remove a multitude of foods from the diet of the child, the single food that is eaten every day in some form or another and craved by the child is completely removed. If other foods are removed and the child continues to eat the trigger food, no amount of diet manipulation will produce long-lasting change. This is a recipe for frustration and the main reason many people decide that eliminating a food doesn't make a difference. This is also the reason that people following an elimination diet often find very little benefit. They remove many of the suggested foods, but because the trigger food is over-consumed, craved, and a family favorite, they decide removing it will be too difficult, and their efforts at adjusting the diet make very little difference to the health or behavior of their children.

By supporting parents to simply substitute another healthy food in place of the one that is responsible for their reactions, their family's diet is changed with very little visible change in the menu. By educating people how to substitute for things such as milk, gluten, nuts, soya, and many other common foods in their normal recipes, the adjustment required by the child is minimized. The child is still able to eat a wide range of other healthy foods and is less likely to feel restricted.

By removing this offending food 100 percent and carefully rotating the other foods that are eaten, children get well. When the over-consumed food is removed, their tastes begin to change, and they are more receptive to eating a wider range of fruits, vegetables, and meats. I tell this to parents all the time, at which point they laugh and reply, "You don't know my child. He has never eaten a green vegetable in his life, and he is eight." I smile and encourage them to give it a try and see for themselves.

The best example I have ever had of this phenomenon is a little nine-year-old boy with autism who had never spoken a word in his life. His diet consisted only of plain wheat pasta and pizza with most of the topping scraped off. After only three weeks of substituting rice pasta and a rice pizza crust, he began to speak in full sentences and eat the fruits and vegetables which he had refused all his life. The transformation for this child was profound.

Following the explanation of some of the tests and diets commonly used to identify food sensitivities by other professionals, you will find a questionnaire to complete. This will help you identify the often hidden trigger food that is the cause of your child's symptoms.

TYPES OF FOOD SENSITIVITY TESTING USED BY OTHER HEALTH CARE PRACTITIONERS

Real-Life Story

Despite reassurances from the doctor that Gabriel is healthy, his parents, Laurie and Rob, are convinced that something must be wrong. They are optimistic that the appointment they have today with the allergist will offer them some answers. It simply isn't normal for a child to be so tired, irritable, and miserable after being so happy only weeks before.

Gabriel entered the world as a quiet, happy, and easy-to-care-for baby. He slept, ate, smiled, and was a huge gift to his parents after their experience with his colicky older sister. Gabriel, however, changed dramatically at the age of two when he had his first dose of antibiotics for tonsillitis. It was as if someone had flipped a switch, and Gabriel became irritable, uncooperative, and complained of tummy aches and being tired all the time. The happy and energetic little boy seemed to disappear overnight to be replaced by a demanding and chronically unwell little guy who is exhausting his parents.

At the encouragement of a friend who is a nurse, Gabriel's mom is taking him to an allergist in hopeful anticipation of finding out if food is creating a problem for her son. After only a few minutes of conversation, the allergist assures Laurie that her son's symptoms could very likely be related to food and he begins a long series of scratch tests. To Laurie's dismay, her child receives over twenty scratches on his arms and back, and he howls throughout the entire procedure. His cries to his mom of "Why are you letting them do this to me?" broke her heart, and she sobs herself as she tries to comfort him through the test. When it was over, the allergist then announced to Laurie that these tests are only about 50 percent accurate for foods and that he wants to place Gabriel on a multiple food elimination diet. Laurie was horrified. Why had he not told her this before he did the test? Why had she not known enough to ask?

The allergist then gave Laurie a list of common foods that are known to be potential allergens and asked her to remove all of these foods from her son's diet for a week and then add them back one food at a time. As Laurie picks up her son and leaves the office, she is overwhelmed, angry, and confused about how to implement the diet she has been given. The foods on the list are the only ones that Gabriel will eat and the ones she serves every day to her family. What will she feed them now? Where will she find the alternatives? Will they fit in her food budget that doesn't have much room for extra expenses? Will all of this work actually find the answer she is looking for?

While there are several types of tests to determine food sensitivities, none of them give accurate information on food intolerances. Laurie's story is a common one where people are given many types of tests that often result in frustration and misinformation. By identifying the trigger food by the process outlined in this book, the cause of Gabriel's problem would be easily identified without these painful tests and overwhelming diet restrictions.

It has been my experience over the last twenty-seven years that one of the reasons food sensitivities are not better understood or identified as the cause of children's symptoms is because the tests most professionals use can be complex, painful, or overwhelming to undertake by most families. I see clients all the time who have sought medical or naturopathic help in identifying a food that might be part of their child's problem but who eventually abandoned the exercise. My process for identifying the hidden, underlying trigger food is medically sound, simple, fully supported, and successful for parents in the midst of their busy lives. I believe that children deserve every chance to realize their full potential, and I know firsthand the power that diet change can make. The process has to be easy for a parent to do in the midst of their already busy lives.

The tests, however, offered both by the naturopathic and the traditional medical communities are valuable and appropriate for some children. For those with anaphylactic reactions to foods, identifying the offender and then removing it completely is essential and should be done under the watchful eye of an experienced allergist. Scratch type tests are also very reliable for inhalant allergies such as pollens, grasses, dust, and chemicals. For most parents, however, facing the possibility of extensive elimination diets, multiple scratch tests, or the trial removals of a long list of common foods feels overwhelming. There are several types of testing that are commonly used to help parents identify foods that might be bothering their children. Below there is a brief description of each one. However, the most complete process for trigger food identification and elimination is the one I have developed and outlined in this book.

Skin tests

Skin tests involve a process where a wide range of potentially offending substances are injected just under the skin of the child. Some physicians use a small scratch procedure, and some inject the substance under the skin with a very small needle. The child then waits in the office for about fifteen minutes, and the injection sites are observed for any signs of swelling or redness that indicate a reaction as a result of the release of histamine. Although very rare, children may also have a severe response with this type of testing, so it should be done in the office of an allergist or doctor who has the appropriate medications and expertise to deal with such a reaction.

This type of testing is very accurate for environmental and airborne substances such as pollen, grasses, or dust but is very inaccurate for food. The redness that denotes a positive reaction is caused by the release of IgE antibodies, and these are only present with true allergic reactions. As was discussed in chapter two, most reactions to food are intolerances rather than allergies. The result is that although the testing appears negative, the child still often has symptoms when the food is consumed. Unfortunately, many parents are told that a certain food is not a problem for their child—despite the fact that they are convinced their child's symptoms are worse when the food is eaten—because these skin tests are normal. This type of testing is also quite inaccurate in babies and very small children, as their level of IgE is still very low.

There is also a skin test that is done by some physicians where a patch is impregnated with the potentially offending food and then applied to the skin for forty-eight hours. This is intended to help identify delayed reactions to foods that may be missed during the shorter period of time used in the scratch test. The patches that are used are currently poorly standardized, so the results are not considered to be consistently accurate. Because it still measures an IgE mediated response, this test also is inaccurate for food reactions due to food intolerances.

Blood tests

The most commonly used tests are the RAST test and the ELISA test. Blood tests are more expensive than skin tests and are usually used for severe sensitivities where it is unwise to expose the person to the offending substance or when there is a severe case of eczema or dermatitis which makes finding a skin test location difficult.

The RAST test involves measuring specific allergic antibodies in a person's blood. The test is slightly more accurate than the skin testing for food, but the results are still difficult to interpret. Like skin tests, blood tests are dependent upon the presence of IgE antibodies to give a positive response. Because many food reactions are not linked to the release of histamine or the presence of IgE antibodies, the food causing the physical symptoms is often missed.

The ELISA tests also measure the presence of IgG antibodies in the blood, and some researchers believe it is an accurate method to identify food intolerances, which are the reactions that are delayed and most common. There are currently very few labs that perform this procedure, and many articles report that there is a wide discrepancy in the results. Because most food intolerances are the result of a localized inflammation in the bowel, this type of testing is not likely to provide much in the way of practical help. If you make a decision to try this test, be sure to have a competent health care professional interpret the results for you in light of your own symptoms. As is true for any medical tests, the results are to be considered in combination with an accurate and complete history, other blood work, and tests that may also be required to get an accurate diagnosis.

One additional concern about blood tests for food sensitivities is the number of home testing kits that are appearing on the market. The Internet is full of companies promising instant identification of your offending foods within a few short days. They send you a kit, have you prick your own finger, and then have you add drops of blood to a tube they send you. You then mail the sample back to them and await your results. Because of the variability of these labs and the procedures that they use, it is not recommended that you attempt to find your answers in this manner. If you want to try the ELISA blood test, many naturopaths have access to reputable labs both in Canada and the US that guarantee the accuracy and standard of their tests. You then have access to the support of the naturopath to appropriately interpret your results.

Multiple food elimination and challenge testing

The determination of foods that may be the cause of your child's symptoms is most accurately achieved by removing foods for a period of time and then reintroducing them. This multiple food elimination method is often used by allergists and naturopaths and is the one undertaken by many of the clients before they come to see me. While removal of the food and then reintroduction of it offers the best chance of identifying the cause of the symptoms, removal of many different foods or foods identified only as common offenders can be difficult and the offending food of an individual child is often missed.

The major drawbacks of this type of approach are that it feels overwhelming to most parents to remove multiple common foods from their family's diet and that it is often poorly supported by the professional who orders it. The parent is given a long list of common food allergens and told to remove them completely from the diet of their child for a week. This usually strikes immediate concern in the parent, as the list always contains all the foods the child and family eat on a regular basis. The diet usually removes dairy, gluten, egg, soya, peanut, corn, seafood, and citrus, which are the ingredients in the diet of almost every child and family. How is a mother to make a school lunch for her child with the foods that are left? Will her child really eat a stir fry or a soup made of vegetables along with rice crackers and blueberries? Most children resist the diet, and many parents abandon the process before they have even begun. If the parent truly is committed to trying to make this work, the parent is often met with roadblocks and frustrations, as they have no idea where to purchase alternative foods such as dairy-free milk, gluten-free bread, or foods that don't contain at least a trace of corn hidden somewhere. Despite the commitment to make it work, the parent often gives the forbidden foods by mistake, and it is impossible to predict the cause of any reactions the child has.

The other challenge that the multiple food elimination diet process often produces is in the method of adding foods back to the child's diet. They are added one at a time, and often the parents are told to feed the child this food three or even four times a day to see if a reaction results. Many children are intolerant to a food—but only if it is consumed in large quantities over a short period of time. When this process is used, many foods cause symptoms and are removed from the diet but could be eaten if they were given in small quantities with spaces of rest in between. As well, many reactions to foods are delayed and do not appear for two or three days. If foods are added back too quickly, it is impossible to determine which food caused the response, and the results are again invalid.

Some physicians are more thoughtful in how they approach this elimination diet and remove only one food at a time. This is much easier to manage for the family and far more likely to enlist the cooperation of the child. I have seen, however, many families where this approach has been tried multiple times, and the food causing the symptoms has not been identified. The reason for this is that the physician is removing foods that are identified in the literature as being the most likely to cause a reaction rather than making the choice based on the individual diet and preferences of the child. Unless the correct offending trigger food is found and removed from the diet, there is usually very little improvement in the child's symptoms.

Other types of testing

There are a number of other, nonconventional types of tests available. Some naturopaths use a machine called a VEGA machine and attempt to identify the offending foods using the flow of electromagnetic energy. This testing has no randomized and double-blind studies to address its accuracy. I have had the testing done, personally, a number of times and found the accuracy to be very good. The testing is highly dependent on the skill of the person performing it and is only useful in conjunction with a full history and interpretation by a health care professional well-educated on food sensitivities. There have been lawsuits related to this testing where people have made treatment decisions based solely on the results rather than considering the results as part of a complete medical evaluation.

The other method of testing commonly used by complementary physicians is kinesiology testing. In this test, the patient holds his or her arm out at right angles to their body, and a second person pushes down with enough effort to push the arm toward the floor. The tester then has the patient hold a food in the area at the base of their neck with one hand, and the other person pushes down on the patient's arm again. The principle idea is that if the food is not tolerated, the patient will not be able to hold their arm up, and the arm will collapse weakly toward the floor with very little pressure. Again, I have tried this type of testing and have found the results very intriguing. I have experienced many instances where, even when the food is disguised, my arm becomes weak when I hold foods that create symptoms for me. This test is also difficult because of the patient's arm becoming weak from overuse or the person who is applying the pressure being inconsistent in their effort. If you want to give this a try, please do not base your decision about whether to eat a food on this test. There are far too many uncontrolled variables to allow it be considered accurate enough for those decisions. It is best to follow the process of eliminating the one food you have identified as the trigger for a period of a month and then challenging it by eating it again. This is the only truly accurate way to identify a food that is creating symptoms.

It is because of the difficulty in identifying the offending foods that most people find their way to see me. I believe that the only accurate way to help a child get well and have the family be successful in changing their diet is to determine the trigger food accurately at the beginning. Once the food has been identified, it is then essential that the family gets the needed support to make the necessary changes and adaptations so the diet is successful.

TYPES OF DIETS COMMONLY USED TO ADDRESS FOOD SENSITIVITIES

The Internet is loaded with quick-fix diets and guaranteed solutions for every ailment and illness known to mankind. In this culture of instant solutions, people often fall prey to these gimmicks because their symptoms are causing so much misery in their lives. My approach to addressing the topic of food sensitivities is a holistic one and is individualized to the diet, health, and lifestyle of each individual client I see. I have seen firsthand how a diet that claims to solve a wide range of health problems fails in a huge number of cases. There is no one diet that works for everyone, just as there is no one lifestyle that we all need to follow. It is only by being treated as an individual and having all the aspects of your life considered before any recommendations are made that successful, sustainable diet changes and lifestyle adjustments are possible.

Below I list a few of the common diets for you to be aware of. I do not endorse any of these diets; although I have seen some people achieve some significant improvement. The opposite is also true, however. I have seen clients who religiously followed a particular diet only to have their health deteriorate. The diet they chose resulted in an overconsumption of a food that was a trigger for that particular person, and they became quite ill very quickly. An individualized approach is the only sure way to remove the appropriate food and regain your health.

Gluten-free/casein-free diet

This diet removes all gluten-containing grains, such as wheat, barley, spelt, oats, and rye and all foods containing any type of dairy products. It is often used by families with an autistic child, as the literature strongly suggests that removal of both gluten and dairy-containing foods can improve the child's symptoms significantly.[21] I have seen clients where it has made difference in their child. My criticism here is that many other foods are now over-consumed, and children who have an issue with eggs or other common foods show no improvement or actually get worse. This diet also results in people over-consuming sugar-loaded baking, as the child reaches often for gluten-free cupcakes, cookies, and sweets that they likely would not otherwise consume. While it is necessary to allow kids to have these tasty alternatives in the beginning, over-consumption of them results in poor nutrition, which does not support their overall health. The extra sugar can also promote the growth of Candida in their bowel and result in a worsening of their symptoms. Also, because my philosophy is to remove the least number of foods from a child's diet in order to make them well, it is very possible that the trigger food for many children is only dairy or gluten, and the removal of both foods in unnecessary.

Specific carbohydrate diet

This diet was developed and extensively studied by Elaine Gottschall, M.Sc., a scientist who lived and worked in both Canada and the United States. It removes all complex, starchy carbohydrates from the diet and uses nut flour as the basis for the baking of cakes, cookies, and muffins. The principle is that complex carbohydrates are difficult to digest when the digestive tract is very inflamed with the result that these foods ferment in the bowel and are responsible for a wide number of symptoms. The literature produced on this diet suggests that it is particularly effective in people with severe inflammatory bowel disease such as ulcerative colitis, Crohn's disease, and irritable bowel syndrome as well as autism.[22.]

My concern with this diet is the same as with the gluten and dairy-free one. The cooking and baking results in the consumption of a huge number of eggs and nuts and these may be poorly tolerated by some people. The diet may be appropriate in terms of the removal of the grains and other starches, but other foods—such as eggs—may also need to be eliminated. I tried this diet myself a couple years ago and become increasingly ill. Through the process, I discovered that consuming many eggs and nuts resulted in a worsening of my symptoms, even though eating the occasional portions of these foods had not been a problem. An individualized approach definitely works better, but if your symptoms are severe, the removal of all the grains from your diet—including rice—may be what is required for a period of time.

Anti-Candida diet

This diet is used for the treatment of an overgrowth in the bowel of Candida Albicans, which is a type of fungus or yeast. Candida is present in the normal flora of our digestive system but can grow out of control with excessive use of antibiotics, hormones, many medications, or stress. This diet is based on the idea that foods that contain large amounts of sugar feed the yeast and allow it to grow out of control. The diet removes all fruits; fermented foods, such as cheeses, alcohol, vinegar, and pickles; moldy foods, like mushrooms and peanuts; sugars of any kind, yeast containing breads and caffeine. Some physicians also remove all the gluten-containing grains. The diet requires strict adherence to this program for at least a month in order to see any improvement.[23.] Many naturopaths also give their patient some type of yeast-killing medicine at the same time to speed up the process.

As with the other diet, what is missing here is an individualized approach. Food sensitivities are one of the major causes of bowel inflammation and thus cause an increase in the yeast population. Unless these foods are removed from the diet, all the other adjustments being made will have little effect. I have seen people struggle through this diet, yet over-consume things like eggs or certain vegetables that are problematic and receive very little benefit for all their effort.

Low-histamine diet

Histamine plays an important role in protecting us from invading organisms and is involved in the regulation of stomach acid, muscle contraction, blood vessel permeability and brain function.[24.] The amount we have in our body varies due to a number of factors. Certain foods we eat contain histamine, and other foods result in the natural release of histamine within our bodies. As well, when the balance of bacteria is altered due to antibiotic use, medications, hormones, or food sensitivities, some of the bacteria that overgrow also produce histamine. This can result in the level of histamine in our bodies surpassing our normal threshold and we develop a wide variety of symptoms.

The symptoms produced often mimic other diseases and allergic reactions, which makes diagnosis of this problem difficult. People may experience runny noses, itching, digestive upset, excessive sleepiness, or headaches. If other types of diet adjustment or medications have been unsuccessful in alleviating symptoms, it is worthwhile giving this diet a try. By decreasing the amount of histamine-containing foods, such as berries, seafood, avocado, tomatoes, or leftover protein foods, the total amount of histamine in the body can be decreased. It is also helpful to address food sensitivities by removing the offending trigger food effort the decrease bowel inflammation and the number of histar producing bacteria in the bowel. Adding probiotics to the diet may also help decrease the number of histamine-producing bacteria, although there is no current research that identifies exactly what balance of organisms is most effective.

The body normally breaks down the histamine in our body using two specific enzymes. These enzymes can be destroyed when the bowel is inflamed and may account for the increase in symptoms during serious digestive disease or with food sensitivities. There is a product on the market called Histame that can be taken when you consume high-histamine-containing foods. It contains one of the natural enzymes that breaks down histamine and can help to decrease the symptoms you experience when you eat these foods. The website for this product that you must buy over the Internet is *www.histame.com*

I have personally had clients develop the symptoms related to histamine intolerance months after the removal of a trigger food from their diet. As they adjusted their eating habits to include healthier and more natural food, they over consumed high histamine foods such as fish, tomatoes, avocado and berries and developed many of the symptoms of a true food allergy. The hives, headache, and itchiness they experienced were not, however, relieved by antihistamines. This provided the clue that perhaps the problem was related to the high histamine foods in their diet and the symptoms were relieved when these foods were removed. It is also important for people facing this challenge to ensure that they take a regular dose of probiotics to help minimize the number of histamine producing bacteria in their bowel.

COMPLETE MEDICAL AND FAMILY HISTORY FORM TO DETERMINE TRIGGER FOOD

Identification of food sensitivities requires a systematic and organized approach. Because the symptoms can be delayed for as long as twenty-four or thirty-six hours after the food is consumed, it is essential that a step-by-step approach is followed. It is important to remember that rarely is anyone bothered by a multitude of foods. Unlike the common practice of removing many foods from the diet and then slowly reintroducing them, I prefer a different approach. When the trigger food is identified and removed completely from the diet, the other foods that may be a small problem are very quickly tolerated again. The common mistake made by many people when undertaking an elimination type of diet is that they remove most of the foods completely, but the trigger food remains because it is the most difficult one to live without. Only by identifying this trigger and removing it completely will the symptoms subside and health be restored.

On the next pages, you will find a history form to fill out. Some of the questions will relate back to those issues that are known to cause food sensitivities discussed in chapter two as well as collect information about your family history and the diet preferences of your child and your family. It is by compiling all of these answers together that the trigger food that is causing the symptoms will become clear. Take time to consider each question carefully and refer back to the answers you gave on the signs and symptoms sheet in chapter one if you need to.

Once you have determined the food, keep reading the rest of the book. It will support you as you make the change work in the real lives of your family.

Questionnaire

Family History

List any symptoms or illnesses that you, your child's other parent, or your child's siblings have had. Refer to the signs and symptom checklist in chapter one so you won't forget anything. Please list them all, even if they do not seem to be connected to food sensitivities or diet.

List any symptoms or illnesses that members of your child's extended family have, including grandparents, aunts, uncles and cousins. Please consider all the items in the checklist in chapter one as well as anything else that might not have been mentioned. Even if you are unsure if a symptom is related to a food sensitivity, include it anyway.

List any foods that are known to cause symptoms in any member of your child's family or extended family.

Effects on infant during pregnancy

When your child was in utero, was the mother sick with any disease or illness?

What, if any, symptoms did your child's mother have during any of her pregnancies that were troublesome?

Did your child's mother drink alcohol or take any type of medications or drugs during her pregnancy?

Did your child's mother ever notice any repetitive behaviors or levels of activity in her unborn child? For example, did he or she always hiccough in the morning or kick wildly after dinner?

Describe any stressful experiences that occurred in the life of your child's mother when she was pregnant.

List any symptoms that you are aware of that were present in the grandmothers of your child when they were pregnant.

Method of feeding

Was your child bottle-fed or breastfed?

Did your child experience bouts of excessive crying, gas, or colic if they were breastfed? List any foods that were consumed by the mother when breastfeeding that were identified as a possible cause.

At what age was your child weaned and what type of drinks were they given next?

What formula, if any, was your child given and when? Please describe any reaction that occurred.

Describe any change in the child's health or behavior when they were weaned.

As an infant, did your child have any specific behavior or health concerns? Examples might be colic, diarrhea, runny nose, excessive fussiness, skin rash, cradle cap, red or pinpoint rash on buttocks, white patches in their mouth, or a diagnosis of a fungal infection either in their mouth or on the buttocks.

Describe the method of feeding and any symptoms that occurred during the infancy of both of your child's parents.

Introduction of solid food

At what age were solid foods first introduced to your child?

List the approximate sequence of foods that were added to your child's diet and indicate how frequently a new food was added.

List any foods that you believe caused any type of reaction in your child, however mild.

List any foods that you are aware of that caused symptoms for your child's mother as a young child.

List any foods that you are aware of that caused symptoms for your child's father as a young child.

Current diet and nutrition

List your child's five favorite foods. These should be foods your child eats almost every day in some form or another. For example, they might drink milk and eat cheese, yogurt, or ice cream and also eat cheese Doritos, cheese Goldfish crackers, or Stone Wheat Thins, which are loaded with milk.

List the foods that your child reaches for when they are tired and stressed.

Identify what you think is your child's absolute favorite food. This is the food that your child reaches for when they are upset and the one that would be most difficult to give up. If your child is old enough, ask what their favorite food is or what food they would eat if they could have as much as they wanted.

Identify any food you believe creates symptoms of withdrawal in your child when it isn't eaten for several hours. The symptoms of withdrawal are usually an exaggeration of symptoms already present in your child such as deterioration in their behavior or an increase in their physical symptoms such as tummy aches or runny nose.

Write a list of the foods that your child would eat in a typical day, including all meals and snacks.

List foods that your child dislikes.

List any foods that you know bother your child and create any type of symptoms, however mild you think they are. Please write beside them the symptoms you believe they produce. Don't forget to refer to the signs and symptoms sheet you filled out and ensure you consider physical, behavioral, and learning symptoms.

List the five favorite foods of your child's mother and the one you believe would be the most difficult for her to give up.

Identify any symptoms your child's mother has that she believes may be connected to any of these foods.

List the five favorite foods of your child's father and the one you believe would be the most difficult for him to give up.

Identify any symptoms your child's father has that he believes may be connected to any of these foods.

List any diet changes that you have already tried with your child and the impact you believe they have had.

List any actions that you took—either on your own or with the support of a health care professional—in an effort to eliminate your child's symptoms. List what you believe to be the outcome of these efforts.

Multiple doses of antibiotics

List any antibiotics that were taken by the mother of your child during her pregnancy and give the reason for the treatment.

List any antibiotics that your child has had along with the symptoms they were meant to treat.

List any antibiotics that were taken by your child's mother while she was breastfeeding.

List any recurrent symptoms that your child's mother has had that have required repeated courses of antibiotics.

List any recurrent symptoms that your child's father has had that have required repeated courses of antibiotics.

Have either parent or your child ever been treated for a fungal infection? What treatment was used, and was it effective?

Has your child ever taken probiotics?

Autoimmune diseases and diseases of the digestive tract

Has anyone in your child's extended family been diagnosed with a disease of the digestive tract? Please list the condition and the relationship to your child.

Does anyone in your child's extended family suffer from an autoimmune disease such as rheumatoid arthritis, ankylosing spondylitis, or systemic lupus? Please list the disease and the person's relationship to your child.

Medications

Is your child, or either of his or her parents, taking any medications that may cause digestive symptoms?

Life stresses

What things in the lives of your child's parents are causing the most significant stress? Do they feel in a position to change any of them? If not, what is preventing them from doing so?

What stresses do you believe are currently impacting your child?

What stresses do you believe have impacted your child in the past?

How do you believe these stresses have impacted your child's health?

(This topic will be covered in depth in chapter five of this book.)

SUMMARY POINTS FOR IDENTIFICATION OF OFFENDING TRIGGER FOOD

Below you will now be asked to take the common threads from your previous answers and place them in the spaces below. Take time to ponder each question and refer back to your answers in the earlier sections of this questionnaire as well as the signs and symptoms sheet you filled out in chapter one. You should notice common threads between your child and their extended family as well as one food that consistently appears as the answer to many of the questions.

The food you will be removing from your child's diet is

1. The food that is craved by several members of your child's extended family and eaten very often.
2. The food that some members of your child's family reach for when they are stressed or over tired.
3. The food that you identified as being a potential cause of symptoms or chronic illness for some members of your child's extended family. If there is more than one food, list them all.
4. The food that is known to produce symptoms in members of child's family that is similar to the symptoms experienced by your child.
5. The food that has been a problem in some form for most of your child's life, even when consumed by his or her mother during breastfeeding or pregnancy.
6. The food that was introduced to your child when they were young that you believe coincided with the beginning of some of their symptoms.
7. The food that you believe has increasingly become a problem for your child following several courses of antibiotics or other medication.
8. The food that your child craves and would find the most difficult to give up.

9. The food that one or both of your child's parents crave and would find the most difficult to give up.

10. The food that your child reaches for when they are tired and stressed or when their blood sugar is low.

11. The food your child eats every day in some form or other unless they are sick.

12. The food your child craves after they are sick as soon as they are feeling better.

13. The food that produces symptoms of withdrawal when it is not eaten for several hours.

14. The food your child may love in one form and hate in another—for example, your child may crave cheese desperately but hate to drink milk.

15. The food that is present in most things your child eats. For example, your child's favorite crackers may be loaded with milk, the bread they love may be cheese bread, they may love cereal as a bedtime snack, the only chips they like are sour cream, they won't eat potatoes unless they are mashed with milk, or they won't eat veggies unless they have a cream-based dip. The common item in all of these foods in dairy products.

16. The food that seems to consistently produce symptoms each time your child eats it. This is the food that you intuitively have "wondered" over the years if it was a problem and often seems to be the one your child has eaten when they complain of feeling unwell.

17. The food you are hoping desperately not to have to remove from your family's diet. This may be because you crave it and can't bear the thought of not having it in the fridge or because it is the only food your child will eat and you are sure they will starve without it!

Based on your answers to all these questions, which food do you believe is the one causing most of your child's symptoms? If you have identified two foods, one of these is more likely to be the cause than the other. Choose the one you believe to fulfill most of the criteria listed above, and begin with this food. It is important to do only one food at a time. As it is impossible to predict how much health and healing you will get from the removal of a food, it is important to try one first and then try the other if some symptoms still persist. The goal is always to remove the least amount of food from the diet possible and still eliminate the bothersome symptoms.

THE FOOD THAT IS THE PRIMARY CAUSE OF YOUR CHILD'S SYMPTOMS IS:

_____

The following chapters will now help you change your child's diet successfully. Don't stop here. Embrace the possibilities and stay committed to giving it a try.

IDENTIFICATION OF THE UNDERLYING TRIGGER FOOD

- Diet change requires a holistic approach. Good educational information must be combined with a proven process to follow and adequate support.
- Traditional allergy skin and blood testing is reliable for food allergies but does not give adequate information about food intolerances. Most food reactions are intolerances, and the only adequate process to determine the offender is removal of the offending trigger food.
- Removal of a single trigger food that is causing symptoms for an individual child most often results in significant improvement in symptoms and avoids the necessity of the removal of multiple foods.
- Removal of the trigger food will support the child to expand his or her food choices, and gradually, your child will be willing eat a wide variety of new and healthy foods.
- The trigger food must be removed from the diet 100 percent for a month, and the other foods in the diet must be rotated to avoid the development of new problem food.

FOOD SENSITIVIITY TESTING

- There are a number of types of food sensitivity testing, but most have a large degree of inaccuracy for food intolerances. Because food intolerances are not the result of the release of histamine, many tradition types of testing are not helpful in diagnosing the offending trigger food. Both skin and many blood tests measure the presence of IgE antibodies and the release of histamine which are not present in food intolerances.

- The types of testing discussed are
  1. Skin testing
  2. Blood tests
  3. Elimination and challenge diets
  4. Vega testing
  5. Kinesiology testing

DIETS COMMONLY USED TO ADDRESS FOOD SENSITIVITIES

- There are a number of common types of diets that are used to help identify and treat food sensitivities. Each of them may offer some advantages, but it is only through an individualized approach that the trigger food is successfully identified and removed. Trying a diet without identifying the offending foods unique to the individual often results in frustration and failure.
- Diets discussed in chapter three
  1. Gluten-free/dairy-free
  2. Specific carbohydrate
  3. Anti-Candida
  4. Low histamine

COMPLETE MEDICAL AND FAMILY HISTORY FORM TO DETERMINE TRIGGER FOOD

- The most accurate way to identify the major offending food and to avoid extensive testing is to complete the questionnaire in this chapter. By considering all aspects of your child's life, including their personal and extended family history, you will be able to identify the major offending food that is causing your child's symptoms.

SUMMARY POINTS FOR IDENTIFICATION OF OFFENDING TRIGGER FOOD

- This section summarizes the answers from all sections of the medical and family history form to determine the trigger food.

CHAPTER FOUR

AM I READY TO CHANGE OUR DIET?

RESISTANCE: A NORMAL RESPONSE TO CHANGE

Even the word *resistance* often conjures up a physical feeling of irritation and pushback. Most of us hate the experience of feeling pushed into doing something we don't want to do, even if we can see that the benefits might be in our own best interest. There is something universal in us all that prefers choosing the path of our choices rather than having others directing them.

What happens, then, when your own resistance gets in the way of making better choices or necessary changes? What happens when your resistance is entrenched in some old and outdated story or belief from your past that is preventing you from having an open mind? What if your resistance is actually keeping you stuck in a situation that needs to change?

We resist change for a multitude of reasons, and all of them may seem valid and reasonable to us at the time. Changing our diet or the diets of our children is no different than any of the other changes we make in our lives.

Often the perceived risk of the change feels greater than any benefit we believe we will achieve, so we make a decision to stay where we are. Our lives may seem comfortable or predictable, even in the midst of challenges, and we often believe that the energy expenditure to change is more than we can manage in the mist of our current situation. The idea of change may feel overwhelming, as we are lost and not sure where to begin. Our lives may already be so stressful that we believe we simply cannot take on one more thing. It is also possible that we may have taken a few small steps toward change and been discouraged. Perhaps we were criticized by some of the people in our lives that matter. We may lack the support around us that we need to stand up with strong boundaries to stick up for the decisions we feel we want to take in service of ourselves and our children. The pressure around us not to change may be greater than we feel we can navigate. We might even convince ourselves that the change we are considering is not wise or based on accurate and valid information, so we are comfortable simply dismissing it without exploring it fully. Healthy skepticism is important, but a closed mind and a refusal to consider information and investigate the possibilities often prevent us from being open to new ideas.

The behaviors of resistance

How do you know when you are stuck in a place of resistance? How would you recognize that you are accepting the status quo, even when it offers significant challenges? How do you know you have given up the idea of considering what you might change?

See if any of the behaviors of resistance listed below are familiar to you. As you consider adjusting the diet of your family, are you using any of these behaviors to justify not taking some type of action?

1. You complain over and over to anyone who will listen to your difficult story, yet immediately reject any ideas or suggestions offered by others.

2. You have resigned yourself to living a life full of challenges, whatever they might be. You may have accepted that parenting is always difficult and that the challenging behavior of your children is simply normal.

3. You may have tried to change but stumbled and then decided it was impossible, so you have simply given up trying anything else.

4. You may actually deny that you have a problem with your children's health, learning, or behavior and believe they are fine—despite comments, suggestions, and feedback from others in your life, such as parents, teachers, or friends.

5. You have adopted the beliefs and ideas from your family rather than make your own decisions about the changes that are right for you. You might feel a desire to change but dismiss the idea quickly when challenged by the ideas or beliefs of others in your life.

6. You might find yourself acknowledging your need to change something but immerse yourself in books, workshops, medical visits, and consultations with people you believe know more about your child than you do. You believe you need to do something but continue to explore and learn rather than actually take a small step toward practical change. You believe there must be a perfect or right step to take and resist doing anything until you are sure what it is.

7. You procrastinate, avoid, and stall over and over. You do plan to change but have to have all your ducks in a row and your life perfectly figured out before you can do it. You haven't figured out yet that this day will never come, as life with children is always unpredictable.

8. You immerse your energy in countless distractions to avoid the real issues of your life. By keeping yourself so busy, you adopt the belief that you don't have time to change. There

is always an issue more pressing than the one you are trying to avoid.

9. You minimize your challenges and often refer to the fact that many others have it worse than you do. You evaluate your issues in light of those of everyone else rather than address your own needs as important and worthy of your time and energy.

10. You simply don't believe that anything will make a difference. You have tried a few things, read lots of books, asked the opinions of others, and have decided it is simply hopeless to try anything more. You decide to simply live with your situation and avoid hoping anything will change. While pushing against life and trying to make things different than they are expends a great deal of worthless energy, finding small, proactive steps to address your challenges increases your sense of power and control in your life and helps you stay connected to hope.

Managing the resistance of your child, family, friends, and professionals

A discussion of resistance wouldn't be complete without addressing the challenge you will face with the resistance offered by others. It might be resistance from your child, other family members, friends, or professionals, and it often makes things difficult for parents attempting to change the diet of their family.

The benefit of addressing food sensitivities on health, learning, and behavior is well-researched and well-documented. There are a multitude of professional articles that support the impact of food on many aspects of our lives, and it is a topic often written about in magazines and newspaper articles. There is also much misinformation, and many people are very resistant to the idea. Some people may be very vocal in the criticism of this topic and minimize the idea of giving it a try. It is my desire and commitment to counter the misinformation that encouraged me to write this book.

1. **Resistance from the child whose diet you want to change:**

If you are experiencing resistance from your child about removing a particular food from his or her diet, the most important thing is your own attitude. If you are ambivalent or lacking in commitment to what you are doing, your child will sense it. The child will quickly learn that if he or she whines or complains long enough, you will give in. *Don't!* Your job is to provide healthy and tasty alternatives so your child won't feel deprived and then to have an expectation they will cooperate. If you try to manage the change by simply giving them carrot sticks all the time, they will not cooperate for long. Model a calm sense of commitment to the plan and resist any outside influence—even from them—to make you cave in. Create some way to reward them for their efforts, and when they slip up, avoid criticism, but insist they get back on track. Do not create a lot of special situations where you allow your child to cheat, or they will embrace cheating themselves when you aren't around.

It is also important to assure your child in the beginning that you are only going to follow the changes for a month, not a lifetime, so they don't anticipate losing their favorite food forever. Tell them you will revisit the topic at the end of the month and will listen to their thoughts on how it went. Be proactive in your solutions, and anticipate events in the life of your child and your family members before they happen. Scrambling at the last minute is usually a recipe for disaster, so plan ahead and keep some appropriate foods in your cupboards and your freezer.

There is a complete section on successfully changing the diet of your child later on in this book, so take time to read it carefully before you begin.

2. **Resistance from other family members and friends**: Comments, criticism, and negative opinions may often be freely expressed on the topic of the impact of food on health and behavior by the well meaning people in your life. It is important that you are strong in your commitment to what you are doing and have planned ahead what to say. There is no need to defend your decision, as it is your life, but it is often helpful to educate your family and speak about the difference you hope it will make.

   If you meet resistance from family members who will be offering food to your child, do your best to educate them on what to do. Give them your child's favorite recipes, buy some snacks to keep at their house, and give them the substitute foods they need to cook for your child. If you find that they continue to sabotage your efforts and feed your child unsafe food, design another plan for your child. It is important that you acknowledge your role as parent and stand firmly behind the decisions you are making. This may mean temporarily avoiding having your child go there for a visit or an insistence that you provide all the food. This is an area where you need strong boundaries and a strong conviction about why you are doing it.

3. **Resistance from professionals:** Some of the most frustrating experiences I have had—both as a mother and a nurse—were in trying to explain the impact of food sensitivities to a wide range of professionals. The topic remains poorly understood, and many professionals from a number of disciplines simply minimize or dismiss the topic. My best advice is to follow your own intuition. Do your homework, and research the topic fully so you understand what you are doing. Ask others who have attempted similar changes, and decide for yourself if it is worth giving it a try. *Do not readjust medications or risk giving your child a food that poses any risk to his or her health, no matter who tells you it is safe. Seek the support of a competent health care professional if you have questions.*

I have witnessed the transformation in the health, behavior, and learning of our four children and our grandchildren, as well as hundreds of clients. The potential to make a difference in your child's challenging symptoms is huge, so I encourage you to give it a try.

Your success will speak for itself, and when you return to your doctor, psychologist, teacher, or behavior specialist and address the significant improvement you have noticed, they won't be able to help but be convinced. The resources section of this book contains a large number of references. You can take a photocopy of a relevant section of one of these resources to your doctor if you feel it would help them understand and support what you are doing.

Questions:

1. As you read the list of behaviors that indicate resistance to change, which ones do you recognize as strategies you often use?

2. If you feel that this strategy is increasing your avoidance of addressing an important issue, what motivating reason can you relate to that will support you to take a small step forward?

3. As you read this list of behaviors that indicate resistance to change, which ones do you recognize as strategies used by your child?

4. If you feel your child is highly resistant to the changes you want to make, what motivating reason could you help them to find that might decrease this resistance and help them cooperate?

5. As you read this list of behaviors that indicate resistance to change, which ones do you recognize as strategies used by other members of your family that will be impacted by the diet change you are considering?

6. Have you found this to be a pattern in your relationship with these people? Has it supported or inhibited you from standing firmly in your decision to make the changes in the past that you have wanted to make?

7. What motivating reason could you help these people to find that might help them be more supportive of your plan?

8. What places of resistance do you anticipate in the other areas of your life and the life of your child?

9. What strategies do you need to employ as you begin to make changes in your family's diet to deal with the resistance and criticisms of others such as teachers, family doctors, counsellors etc.

Resistance—where does it come from?

Resistance is often created by outside influences, and they have an impact on your willingness to take risks and make changes for yourself. The opinions and influences of others often play a big role in your willingness to change. If you examine your own resistance, you will often find places where your excuses are based on things that make you afraid or doubt your own abilities. Unless you actually change things in your environment or cultivate new habits, your old, default stories and intentions become the compass that guides your decisions. As the saying goes, "To be different, you have to do different."

Here is a brief summary of the topics that will be covered in chapter five that influence both your willingness and ability to make changes in some aspect of your life. Chapter five contains questions on each of these topics to help you identify how each of these issues will affect your ability to change the diet of your family.

1. **Your definition of health for yourself and your family:** If you don't feel there is a problem with the health or behavior of your family, you will be resistant to making any type of changes. Even if others tell you there is a problem,

you won't agree and thus won't attempt to do anything differently.

2. **The amount of stress in your life:** Stress plays a big part in your willingness to change. Excessive stress interferes with your ability to problem-solve and prioritize the tasks of your life, and anything extra feels overwhelming. Stress often produces fatigue and exhaustion, so there is little energy left to take on something new.

3. **Your past experiences with change:** If you have tried to make changes in other areas of your life and have been unsuccessful, you are often more resistant to taking on the risk of making new ones. Conversely, positive experiences with change in your past often make you more willing and resourceful in taking on the risk of something new.

4. **The connection of your motivation to something you value:** You embrace changes only when you believe they will offer something that really matters to you. You will actively resist any change that doesn't appear to offer something that will make significant improvement in some aspect of your life.

5. **The balance and priorities of your busy life:** If your life contains so many obligations and commitments that you barely have time to breathe, you will be very resistant to adding more things to your "to do" list. Rather than focusing on what really matters, you are caught up in a huge whirlwind of tasks, and there isn't any energy or room to add something more.

6. **The impact of your old stories and beliefs:** The beliefs you hold about yourself impact your ability to feel confident enough to take risks and embrace change. If you have had positive role models who encouraged you to make empowering choices, you are more likely to find active steps to take. If you doubt your abilities and don't believe you have what it takes, you will often be very resistant to take risks and address the challenges in your life.

7. **Your ability to set healthy boundaries:** You often experience resistance to change because of the opinions and thoughts of others. Even when you believe something is right for you, it is common to give in to the ideas of others and allow them to walk over your personal boundaries. If you allow others to have significant influence over your choices, you will be reluctant to change anything that is not in alignment with what those people think.

8. **Your ability to move past your own doubts and saboteuring voices:** We all have internal, critical voices that are more than pleased to insert doubt into our thoughts as soon as we even ponder making a change. The voices are often familiar ones from your past, and the doubt they create is often enough for you to be resistant to change.

9. **Your willingness to ask for help:** Change is often difficult, and you benefit from the help and support of others. Many people fail in making the changes they want in their lives because they have a belief that they must go it alone. After trying a few times on their own, most people simply give up and are resistant to trying again rather than enlisting the help and support of others.

10. **Your willingness to address issues related to your own health:** This is one of the most common areas of resistance I see in all my clients. Changing the diets of their children most often means taking a cold, hard look at their own lives and their own health. You may need to adjust your own diet or finally face a challenge in your own life that you have been avoiding. Sometimes this concept feels so difficult that people create elaborate excuses and avoid addressing the issues of their children.

STAGES OF CHANGE

There are many books and articles on the steps and stages of change.[25.] In the end, we all change when we are internally motivated to do so. We are either so uncomfortable where we are or are so motivated to get something we value that we are willing to take on the risk and discomfort of changing.

The stages of change are offered here for the purpose helping you notice where you are in respect to the changes in your own life. The stage you are at will vary for each area of your life that is facing a change. While you may embrace the idea of a change in your job, you may be very resistant to the idea of making some changes in your struggling marriage. We often focus the changes we make on the ones that are easy and continue to avoid the changes that feel difficult. Remember, as well, that your child may be at one stage of change, and you may be at another, so you will have to be creative in designing a plan that honors the needs of you both.

Following the description of these stages there are some questions to help you identify which of these stages best identifies where you and your child are with respect to your readiness to make changes in your diet.

Stage one: I don't have a problem.

In this stage, you are not even considering the idea of changing something in your life. You are resistant to the thoughts and ideas of others and actively avoid conversation on the topic. You have arguments to counter anything they say and are committed to maintaining the status quo. You are comfortable where you are, even if others don't see how that is possible, and you are not searching for anything else. Your resistance to change is so strong that you are impossible to move.

At this stage, you are not entertaining any ideas at all related to adjusting your diet or the diet of your child. You are resistant to any ideas offered by anyone and rarely engage in conversation on the topic.

Stage two: If I change, will it be worth the effort?

In this stage, you are beginning to be uncomfortable with something in your life but aren't yet sure if the benefits of a change would be worth it. You are pondering the ideas and possibilities of what you might change and are on a bit of a teeter-totter as you go up and down with the ideas. You are slightly more open and receptive to the ideas of others, although you also quickly latch onto ideas that focus on the risks and negative impact of a change. You may fluctuate for a while between this stage and the previous one as your discomfort in your life shifts. When you experience a negative impact from your behavior, your incentive to consider adjusting your life often increases.

In this stage, you are pondering now and then if changing your child's diet might work but are still easily influenced by the negative thoughts and ideas of others. In those moments when the impact on you or on your child is significant, your incentive increases. You may anticipate a sense of loss for the foods you believe may be the cause and anticipate grieving for the special foods you enjoy if they were removed.

Stage three: I really need to do something about this.

This is the stage when the discomfort you are feeling and the impact on your life have increased to the point where you can't tolerate it any longer. You are now motivated to change—whatever it takes.

You begin actively collecting information, seeking out resources, and looking for ideas of what to do. You sort through what you have learned and begin to create a plan. At the same time, you may experience some confusion and anxiety, as the road ahead still seems cloudy and uncertain.

This is the place where you are willing to explore the possibility of diet change because of the symptoms your child is experiencing. You seek out resources on the topic and find it helpful to hear the stories of other parents. You are aware that there is much to learn, and sometimes, feeling overwhelmed by it all, you slide back to stage one or two for a while. Your resistance to change, however, is often balanced by the discomfort you feel in your situation. As you create a plan that feels possible and design the support you need to make it work within your own day-to-day life, your motivation increases, and you begin to take the first active steps to address the challenges you are facing.

Stage four: I can do this . . . I think.

This is the stage of precarious change. Once you begin to give it a try, you are hoping to see the benefits right away. You need the reinforcement that your efforts are making a difference, or you may quickly slide back into a stage of discouragement. You may doubt that your plan is going to work, or you may fall prey to the criticisms of others. This is the stage—along with stage three—where you must take time to find adequate support and help. You must address proactively all those places where you anticipate you may stumble and add strategies to address them in your plan. If you rush too quickly and impulsively into making a change without adequate planning, your chance of success is low. In order to find sustainable and successful change, it is important to include supportive strategies in your plan.

This stage is the one where most people stumble. It is the stage where, if the diet changes don't produce dramatic and immediate results, people doubt that the idea is going to work at all. It is common for people to quickly abandon the idea as too much work for too little benefit. They don't give it long enough to work. This is the area where I direct most of my support with my clients and the reason for all the coaching sections in this book. Without a strong, realistic plan that addresses all aspects of the lives of the family members and the child, the chances of success are limited. This is reflected in the stories I often hear of people who, in their words, "gave it a try, and it didn't work." They didn't plan well enough, didn't include all aspects of their lives in their plan, and didn't have adequate support as they implemented it. Success is only possible when the challenges of the child and his or her family are addressed in a holistic manner.

Stage five: I can do it, and it makes a difference.

A comprehensive and holistic plan has been created; you feel well-supported in your change and are now feeling successful. Your efforts are being rewarded, and you begin to see a change in the symptoms you are hoping to address. You begin to experience a sense of relief that the stressful situation is getting better, and begin to connect to hope. Some of the things you need to do feel difficult but you are able to quickly connect to the benefits and stay motivated to continue. You have safe places to go for information and support and look forward to life feeling a little easier. You begin sharing your story with others in the hope that they may also give it a try. You are able to counter the doubt expressed by others with conversation about the difference it has made in your life and are less likely than in other stages to be influenced by their opinions.

This is the stage where you begin to trust in your ability to make sustainable change in your child's diet. You can see the benefits both for your child and yourself and feel motivated to continue. You are anxious to share your experience with others and can see how many of your friends are facing similar issues with their children. You are at risk, however, of trying to promote others to change and experience the benefits you have found but meeting with resistance and doubt, as they are still back in one of the earlier stages of change. Your best strategy is to simply lead by example and allow your child's newfound health and behavior to speak for themselves.

Stage six: Oops! I slipped up.

As is human nature, we rarely make perfect changes in our behavior. Some outside pressure, internal stress, or feeling of being fed up with it all inevitably appears, and you slip off the wagon. While you can stay motivated most of the time, sometimes you simply can't find the energy to be bothered. You revert back to your old behaviors and let yourself off the hook from needing to try so hard. If this happens, it is important that you reconnect quickly to your motivations to change and remind yourself of the difference the change has made in your life. Rather than stay stuck in the old, familiar places, you quickly pick yourself up and get back on track. You may need to design some additional support or shift things in your life to make the change more sustainable, but you are committed to making it work. Sometimes, however, if the outside stress or pressure is too much, you can actually slide all the way back to denial and return to your old behaviors all over again. You will only change back when the amount of discomfort you experience increases again or you connect to the price you have paid for not sustaining the change.

Another common place where people stumble in adjusting the diet of their children is when something unexpected happens. This may be a huge family dinner or a birthday celebration at school that you weren't expecting, and the idea of finding alternatives feels simply too much. You convince yourself that a little of the forbidden food won't matter, and you make an exception to your rule. Sometimes the impact is very small, and you arrive at a decision that cheating now and then is something your child can tolerate. Sometimes the consequences are big, and your child becomes very unwell; you decide that the impact wasn't worth it, and you will make another choice next time. Whatever the physical impact, it is important to consider the impact your decision has on your child. While allowing them to choose for themselves is an important coping strategy in helping them stay on the diet, the behavior you model is important. If you minimize the importance of staying on the diet and allow your child to cheat often, they will also minimize the importance of eating the right foods. They will follow your lead and remind you when they cheat that you allowed them to cheat before. It is better to help your child have a voice in how you will adapt to a situation to make it work than to simply cave in because you aren't up to the challenge of finding another way.

Stage seven: I will change because our lives will be better.

This is the stage where you have accepted that the changes you have made are working, and the payoff is worth the effort it takes. You slip back now and then, but quickly return to your motivation and commitment to make the change a sustainable part of your lifestyle. It isn't a topic of focus or extensive conversation and has simply become part of the way you live your life. The benefits are easy to see, and they make a difference in your life that matters to you. You happily share your story with others and are not influenced by their opinions or ideas on what you are doing. You are convinced of the benefits for yourself and have no desire to return to your old behaviors.

With respect to the diet of your family, you have embraced this new way of eating as normal. It is rarely a topic of conversation, and you have moved on to the other important issues of your life. You easily incorporate the diet in your weekly grocery shopping and meal preparation and have developed a repertoire of great menu alternatives. The benefit to your children and your family is so significant that you no longer even consider the idea of going back to the old way of eating. Your life feels less challenged and less stressed now that some of the troublesome symptoms have improved, and you connect to a sense of gratitude that changing the diet of your family has made such a difference. If you or your child occasionally choose to eat the offending food, you quickly are reminded of the consequences and return immediately to eating the right foods again. You are rarely impacted by the thoughts and ideas of others on your diet and are more likely to happily share your successes and the difference the new diet has made in your lives.

Questions:

As you read about these stages of change, which one best identifies where you are now in respect to changing the diet of your family?

If you are in the first two stages, what long-term benefit could you connect to that might increase your motivation to address your child's food sensitivities?

As you read this list of stages, which one best identifies where you believe your child is in respect to changing his or her diet?

If your child does not seem to understand why you think a diet change would be helpful, what consequence or change in their life situation could you help them see that might increase their motivation?

If you have other people or professionals in your life that will be impacted by this change in diet, what stage do you believe they are in?

What strategies might you employ if you sense a great deal of resistance from them with respect to the changes you want to make to help them be more supportive?

STAGES OF GRIEF AND LOSS IN LIFESTYLE CHANGES

Movement through the stages of change is often accompanied by an emotional response. The stages of grief and loss described by Dr. Elizabeth Kubler-Ross match very well this human response to change. Dr. Elizabeth Kubler-Ross describes five stages people experience while dealing with the loss of a loved one; denial, anger, bargaining, depression and acceptance.[26.] These stages have also been used by many others to describe the response we all have to a loss of any kind. They are best thought of, however, as a process rather than linear stages. We all tend to move forward and then back through the stages and may even bypass one all together.

While comparison of these stages to the topic of food sensitivities and diet alterations may seem odd at first, the process bears many similarities. Because food-related activities are a major part of our lifestyle, necessary changes in our usual habits are viewed as a significant stress and with a feeling of loss. The process we go through to eventually live with these restrictions progresses at different rates for different people. Some find it easy to make major alterations in lifestyle by going cold turkey, while others require more time to come to grips with the idea. Neither way is right, but both simply reflect each individual's way of coping.

Many societal rituals revolve around food, so the prospect of altering the diet or lifestyle of a child or your family can feel overwhelming. What will my child do if they can't eat the cake and ice cream at the birthday party? How will I tell my friends that we can't eat the meal they have planned when they invited our family for dinner? The way we adapt to these situations is influenced by many factors, and discussion of this process of adaptation helps us realize we are neither alone nor unique in finding it difficult.

As your life unfolds and other challenges and responsibilities appear, the journey of changing the diet of your family or addressing other issues can become more challenging. The doubt expressed by a grandparent or the dismissal of your efforts by a doctor can send you reeling back to the stages of denial and anger—just when you thought you were finally making progress. However, by the same token, unexpected support and encouragement may also appear and help you find more commitment to the journey you are on. An article in the local paper or a story on the evening news might just be the next piece of support you need to persevere in what you are doing.

When parents are altering the diet of a child, it is also common for both parent and child to be at different stages, with each of them experiencing different challenges and frustrations. This requires much patience on the part of the parent with loads of space offered for the feelings of the child. While a mother may fully embrace and accept the changes, a child may be angry and uncooperative with the new diet. Other family members may also be impacted by the diet changes and thus may also experience frustrations and anger as they are forced to give up foods they love because of the needs of someone else.

Whatever your journey, it is all okay. There is no right way to feel and no right time to feel it. The journey calls for loads of grace for yourself, your child, and your family. If you hit a hurdle, relax and look for a positive step to reconnect to what you are doing and why you are doing it. If you experience a success, celebrate wildly, and help your child to do the same. If you find a great restaurant with delicious and safe food, go often. If you find a healthy and delicious cookie recipe that works, make it often. If you go to a birthday party and it is a disaster, learn from it, and figure out something better to try next time. Ride the roller coaster journey with all its ups and downs, and know that no stage is permanent.

At the end of this section you will find a few questions to help you identify what stage you may currently be in with regard to the diet changes you are making. Remember, however, that these stages change as you adjust to a new way of living.

Denial—my child doesn't have a problem.

Real-Life Story

> Johnny is an active three-year-old who hardly ever sleeps. Even as a baby, he was wakeful and fussy, and his exhausted parents still haven't had a stretch of more than six hours of sleep. He had colic as a baby, and his first ear infection was at two months of age. The antibiotics gave him terrible diarrhea, and he was miserable. He had two more infections between two and six months, and then the story became much worse. Johnny was breastfed until he was six months of age and then switched over to a cow's milk-based infant formula. He then developed eczema on his face and arms, and his bottom became perpetually red. As he began to crawl and then walk, he never, ever stopped. He was always pulling, pushing, banging, shouting, and crying, and his parents were exhausted. His ear infections increased, and it seemed as though a new one reappeared as soon as the antibiotics were finished. Their friends avoided play dates with Johnny because he was so pushy and the family began to notice this distancing from their friends. They loved their little boy and simply chose to believe he was active and busy for his age but that there was no other problem. After all, didn't every child get sick this often? They mentioned it to their doctor but were reassured that Johnny was just an active little boy.

The story is even more difficult now as Johnny's parents have just placed him in preschool. Almost every day he pushes the other kids or grabs their toys, despite his parents' repeated efforts to teach him to share. He is aggressive toward the other children and is quickly becoming isolated. He rarely gets invited to birthday parties, and his recurrent illnesses keep him cooped up at home for extended periods of time.

Johnny's parents are in denial about his problem. When others try to offer unsolicited advice, the parents' response is anger and dismissal of their comments. It is only when Johnny's symptoms impact their life in a way that forces them to take the problem seriously that they will begin to search for some answers.

The period of time between identification of a health, behavior, or learning problem and the time when some type of corrective action begins is individually variable. Because these challenges have such a wide range of normality, identifying that there is, in fact, a problem that needs a resolution may take a great deal of time. Parents may be very resistant to the suggestions or comments of others about their child and simply choose to dismiss what is being said. They also may adopt the rational that it is "just a stage" and trust that their child will simply outgrow the problem down the road. This attitude can also be reinforced by some professionals who may minimize the challenge and cause confusion for parents. Whatever the reason, parents are stuck in the early stages of change and are resistant to taking any type of action.

The list of things that can jar a parent from their stage of avoidance and denial to some type of action is endless. It might be the persistent feedback from the school or daycare that their child is simply unmanageable or struggling in some significant way. It might be that their home environment has become so difficult and stressful, they simply can't go on any longer without finding some relief and respite. It might be a chance article in a magazine, the story of a friend's child, or a book title that calls to them as they walk by a display at a local bookstore.

Whatever the motivator, they are jarred out of their complacent sense of avoidance and forced to come face-to-face with the reality that their child has a problem that needs to be addressed.

Anger—why is this happening to us?

Real-Life Story

> Susie is the mom of ten-year-old George, who is intolerant to both dairy and soya. He has been on the diet for two months over his summer vacation and has shown significant improvement in both his disposition and his ability to focus. Both Susie and George are pleased with the improvement and plan on continuing the diet when school returns in September. George has just been invited to a birthday sleepover by his friend, and he is excited to spend a night with friends whom he hasn't seen all summer. Susie phones the mother of the boy having the party and learns that the food being served is pizza and ice cream cake for dinner and buttermilk pancakes for breakfast. Immediately, she panics and is worried—both about what George will say and how she will manage the problem. She can feel herself becoming angry and resentful that other kids don't seem to have this problem. Why is it happening to her family? Hasn't she done her best to feed them well all their lives? When she tells George about the food, he has a fit and immediately throws his books on the couch and announces he won't be going. He shouts that he is tired of being different and hates the whole thing.

Feeling angry at the concept of having your child feel different and being resentful of the extra work involved in adjusting your family's diet is normal. Even when the changes you have made have improved your child's health, there will continue to be some days when the whole thing feels irritating and frustrating. When this happens, take a break. Go out to dinner, call a friend, take a bath, and disconnect from it for a few minutes. If you are conscientious about planning ahead and already have healthy and delicious alternatives in your cupboards, you will successfully weather these storms without giving in or giving up.

This stage exemplifies the frustration and difficulty that people encounter in making major lifestyle changes. This experience is the same for people attempting to stop smoking, people diagnosed with heart disease who must dramatically change what they eat, and people attempting to remove a food from their diet that they believe is causing undesirable symptoms. Because the task feels difficult, people readily become frustrated and angry when repeatedly faced with problems and are stuck in the early stages of change. When their child is invited to a birthday party or a sleepover, they find the task of providing him or her with safe but acceptable treats very difficult. Their anger may be directed at the doctor, the child, or even themselves, and this increases the stress of an already difficult situation. The child may also feel anger at being forced to be different and may lash out at their parents, believing they don't really understand their frustrations.

This stage may persist for an extended period of time, with some situations causing major angry outbursts on the part of both parent and child. It is also common in this stage for people to be influenced by and resentful of the doubts and criticism offered by others. During this stage, cheating is common, as it is seen as a form of retaliation and a way of gaining control over a frustrating situation. When the connection between the cause and the problem becomes clear, the anger will dissipate to be replaced by positive, thoughtful solutions. When both the child and parent recognize that they are happier and healthier when the child adheres to the diet, they will replace their anger with constructive solutions to make the lifestyle adjustments easier.

Bargaining—I'm sure we'll only have to eat this way for a while.

Real-Life Story

Matthew and Joan are busy, working parents with two school-aged boys, age seven and nine. Both boys were healthy toddlers but began to have trouble at school when they got to grade one. They had trouble focusing, and they seemed to catch every bug that went around. Sean, now age seven, has just developed exercise-induced asthma and is struggling with reading at school. He seems to be in a dream world a lot of the time, and his parents and teachers are always nagging him to hurry up. His brother, Stephen, age nine, is a highly energetic and athletic boy. He excels in sports and absolutely hates sitting still for anything. His teachers are concerned about his inability to focus, and he is beginning to have trouble getting along with his peers. He is also wetting the bed at night, which he finds devastating as it is preventing him from having sleepovers with his friends.

Matthew and Joan have decided to take the whole family off dairy products and food additives. They realize that over the last few years, they have been eating more fast food that was dairy-based and full of food dyes and chemicals. The boys seem to be improving quickly and the family, as a whole, is beginning to feel better. Stephen has stopped wetting the bed and both boys seemed better able to focus, learn, and cooperate.

Just as everyone is feeling encouraged and the school is supportive of the changes the family has been making, sports day appears on the calendar. It is a big event at the school, and the best part for the kids is the treats that are offered. Unfortunately, however, most of them are loaded with milk and additives. Matthew and Joan make a decision to let the boys have a few treats. After all, haven't they been on the diet for two months and done a great job? Surely a few treats won't matter just this once. Perhaps the boys have even outgrown the problem, and the family can return to eating their favorite foods now and then.

This stage of bargaining is also normal, and people often return to it over and over. After being "perfect" on the diet for a while, most people try and convince themselves that a little of the offending food here and there probably won't matter. While it is true that sometimes tolerance is dose-related, it is likely that regular consumption of the trigger food will always result in symptoms.

Unlike the previous stages, this stage is characterized by a feeling of hope and possibility in both the child and his or her family. If the family sticks to the diet and the child's health, behavior, or school performance improves, everyone feels encouraged, as their efforts are being rewarded They cooperate with the restrictions, as they actually see the benefits, but convince themselves that these changes will only be temporary. By placing a limit on the length of time they believe the restrictions will be necessary, the undertaking feels manageable. This strategy is helpful and actually what I encourage people to do in the beginning, as it offers a chance to simply "try it out" and see if it makes any difference. However, once the month is up, honest conversation and an accurate assessment of what has really happened is necessary. Has anything changed? Has it changed enough to make it worth continuing on? Does the family need to try some other food? Did they replace the food to be avoided with an over-consumed alternative the child will have a problem with? Did they truly do it 100 percent, or did they cheat a little here and there so they never really experienced the full benefits of what might be possible? Many people convince themselves that a little bit here and there won't hurt and again push the limit and begin to cheat. When this behavior produces symptoms, they may again return to the stages of denial and anger as a result of their frustration.

Depression—we might have to eat like this forever.

Real-Life Story

Ashley is a sixteen-year-old girl who used to consider herself overweight, unattractive, and an outcast in her peer group at school. She moved to a new high school in grade nine and found it difficult to make friends. She had always struggled in school and found it even more difficult after the move, as the curriculum was different. Her complexion broke out, and she found herself hibernating at home most of the time when she wasn't at school. Although she was a good athlete when she was younger, her extra few pounds made her fearful of participating in any of the teams or activities at her new school.

With the support of her parents, Ashley realizes that her diet is contributing to her health, weight, and emotional issues. She has decided to remove all the gluten-containing bread, buns, and cookies she was eating from her diet to see if it will help. Within a few short days, Ashley has begun to feel better. Her mood is improving, she has lost a few pounds, and her complexion is now improving. She is elated and committed to remaining on this diet.

Ashley had been doing well until Friday night when she was invited to go with a new friend she had made to a movie and dinner. She rationalized to herself that a little bit of pizza and pie wouldn't matter much but soon discovered she was wrong. She felt bloated and uncomfortable for several days afterwards and found herself dropping down again into feelings of being worthless and in despair.

Ashley is disappointed and discouraged that she has so little room in her new lifestyle for those old, familiar comfort foods. She really loves how she feels when she eats what she knows is healthy for her but often finds it very difficult to cope in social situations when her friends are eating the foods she no longer can have.

Ashley's story is common and demonstrates what happens when people realize that the adjustments they have made in their diets are not quick or temporary fixes. These changes are lifelong ways of eating in order to be healthy, and there is often a sense of loss and sadness when people realize this.

It may seem odd that after the positive bargaining stage, a stage labeled depression might follow. While bargaining is characterized by a feeling that the diet changes are temporary, this stage is brought about by the realization that some diet restrictions and lifestyle changes may need to become permanent ways of life. Giving up the large quantity of sugar or junk food consumed by many of us or removing common foods such as milk or wheat feels like a major undertaking and one that is viewed with sadness. As the benefits continue to become evident, the parents and child will eventually progress to the final stage of acceptance, where they will embrace the changes as worth the effort and simply incorporate them into their regular lives. In the meantime, however, there is a sense of sadness at what appears to be the daunting task of finding ways to make these changes a sustainable way of life.

Acceptance—we can do this, and it is worth it.

Real-Life Story

Jason is a twenty-one-year-old university student who has recently moved into an old house with three other friends. He will be cooking for himself and is excited at the idea of being free of university cafeteria food. He has done his best in his first two years of school to stick to the dairy—and gluten-free diet that helped him stay well as a child, but it wasn't always easy. The macaroni and cheese sometimes was the only appetizing choice in the cafeteria, and besides, he longed for that old favorite from his childhood. As he slowly slipped more and more off his diet, he noticed some of his old symptoms beginning to appear. Jason's acne began to return, and he had put on ten pounds in two years. He was aware of feeling more tired than he should and often fell asleep when he was trying to study. He was doing okay but certainly wasn't as healthy or energetic as he was when he lived at home.

Jason embraced the opportunity of shopping and cooking for himself and found many of the familiar brands from home when he went shopping. He stocked his cupboards with healthy and safe alternatives in order to manage those late-night cravings when he was studying and ignored the pizza and nachos left around the house by his roommates.

As his diet shifted, so did Jason's health and he again remembered what it was like to feel well. The better he felt, the more he remembered, and the better choices he made. His friends and his girlfriend noticed a big change in him and acknowledged that he was a much happier guy when he ate well. His roommates were so impressed with the change in him that they, too, began to pay more attention to what they ate. The boys began to cook together and whip up healthy stir-fries and pots of chili rather than eating fast food and eggs. Jason was again connected to the reason his mom helped him to change his diet as a child and remembered that it was well worth the effort.

Even though Jason had slid off the healthy diet he ate as a child, he returned to eating better when his old symptoms began to return. Because he remembered what it was like to feel well, he was better able to make choices to regain his health. As he realized the significant impact this diet had, he found a renewed commitment to make it a permanent way of life.

Progression to the stage of acceptance signifies that the parents, the child, or both have been able to incorporate the diet restrictions into the fabric of their everyday lives and embrace a willingness to change. While they may mourn the loss of favorite foods, they believe that the benefits of the diet outweigh the difficulties. The topic ceases to become one of recurrent conversation and is less likely to result in outbursts of anger and frustration. Because the body begins to heal, occasional cheating may be tolerated, and a previously difficult food may be eaten on special occasions. There will be foods, however, for which tolerance never returns; they will always produce some type of undesirable symptoms. By remembering to rotate healthy foods in a four-day cycle, ensuring the child gets enough rest and exercise, and helping him or her keep the stresses of life in check, your child will be able to lead a healthy and happy life and maximize his or her potential—a true gift to the child and the goal of parenthood.

Questions:

As you read through the stages of grief and loss, which one best addresses how you are feeling at this moment?

What clues will enable you to quickly identify which stage of grief you are in as your response changes?

As you read through the stages of grief and loss, which one best addresses how you believe your child is feeling at this moment? If they are old enough, take time to ask them.

What clues will enable you to quickly identify which stage of grief your child is in as their response changes along the way?

What grief responses have you noticed in other members of your family or extended family as they try and adjust to the changes?

What supportive strategies can you employ for yourself, your child, or other family members to help everyone be patient and accepting of these stages as you experience them?

CHAPTER 4 HIGHLIGHTS

RESISTANCE—A NORMAL RESPONSE TO CHANGE

- Behaviours of resistance.
- Managing the resistance of your child, family, friends and professionals.
- Resistance—where does it come from?

Your readiness to change is influenced by many factors. Unless you address these in a holistic approach, it is very difficult to sustain the change you are hoping to make. The issues that most often influence the ability to change your family's diet are listed below and are covered in depth in chapter five

1. Your definition of health for yourself and your family
2. The amount of stress in your life
3. Your past experiences with change
4. The connection of your motivation to something you value
5. The balance and priorities of your busy life
6. The impact of your old stories and beliefs
7. Your ability to set healthy boundaries
8. Your ability to move past your own doubts and saboteuring voices
9. Your willingness to ask for help
10. Your willingness to address issues related to your own health

STAGES OF CHANGE

- Readiness to change varies depending on the circumstances, and there are seven stages we move through in order to be successful. Following this section there are questions to help you identify which stage of change best represents where you and your family are as you consider a diet change. These stages are:

Stage one: I don't have a problem.

Stage two: If I change, will it be worth the effort?

Stage three: I really need to do something about this.

Stage four: I can do this—I think!

Stage five: I can do it, and it makes a difference.

Stage six: Oops! I slipped up.

Stage seven: I will do this because our lives will be better.

GRIEF AND LOSS

- As we move through the stages of change, we experience emotional reactions to what is happening. The stages of grief and loss apply to diet change, because food is far more than just what we eat. Changes in diet can result in significant feelings of loss. These stages are not linear, and different members of your family can be in different stages at the same time. There are questions in this section to identify which stage best represents your response and the response of your family members to diet change.

  The stages are:

  Denial

  Anger

  Bargaining

  Depression

  Acceptance

CHAPTER FIVE

HOW CAN I GET PREPARED SO I WILL SUCCEED?

Connecting to what motivates you and what will support you to successfully make the necessary diet changes has a huge impact on your long term success. No amount of knowledge will be helpful if you are so overwhelmed at the concept of change that you retreat into old habits or let the voices of doubt cause you to quit. By taking the time to address your whole life—the stresses, challenges, and places of success—you will be better prepared to tackle the job of changing the diet of your family.

THINGS THAT INFLUENCE YOUR ABILITY TO MAKE SUCCESSFUL CHANGES IN YOUR LIFE

As introduced in chapter four, there are ten issues that can create resistance and thereby have a profound impact on your willingness and ability to change. In this chapter you will have an opportunity to explore the areas in your own life that are most likely to create obstacles to your success in adapting the diet of your family. Each of the topics below has some questions that will help you focus on your own specific areas of challenge. They will also help you celebrate your strengths and develop ways to use these abilities to maximize your success in adapting to the changes. As you read through this section, you will likely notice that one or two of the topics seem particularly relevant to your own situation. Do these ones first as managing the most pressing issues will often decrease the impact of other challenges. For example, if your family life is over busy and you are juggling too many things on your calendar, addressing this issue, alone, will necessitate you dealing with your stress level, asking for additional support, and creating healthy boundaries. One small change can thus have a big ripple effect.

The topics in this section are as follows:

Your definition of health for yourself and your family
The amount of stress in your life
Your past experiences with change
The connection of your motivation to something you value
The balance of your busy life
The impact of your old stories and beliefs
Your ability to set healthy boundaries
Your ability to move past your own doubts and saboteuring voices
Your willingness to ask for help
Your willingness to address issues related to your own health

If you would like to purchase the workbook that contains all the questions from this book, go to my website at *www.foodsensitivechildren.com* for information. You will also be able to find additional resources and types of support listed there.

YOUR DEFINITION OF HEALTH FOR YOURSELF AND YOUR FAMILY

Real-Life Story

Alex comes running through the door from school and thrusts a notice into his mother's hands. "Guess what?" he shouts. "We're going on a school camping trip. Can I go? Please?" Alex's grade seven class is celebrating their graduation from elementary school with a camping trip to a local campground. Alex's mom can feel his excitement, but she is overcome with worries and hesitates before giving him an answer. Alex doesn't know how to swim, and she worries about him being close to the water. His repeated ear infections have prevented him from taking swimming lessons, and he is barely able to float without a life jacket. Alex has had ear infections since he was a baby, and his mom keeps a bottle of Amoxicillin in the fridge so she can treat them quickly. Alex also has mild asthma that is well-controlled, but she worries about his level of fitness. He is slightly overweight, and their family is not physically active, so she wonders if the hikes they have planned for the camping trip will be too strenuous for him. The biggest hurdle, however, is Alex's bladder. He continues to have an irritable bladder like his dad did at his age and still occasionally wets the bed. His mom is well aware of the humiliation this would cause her son. What is she going to do?

Alex's mother is now feeling guilty that she didn't seek medical help for his problems earlier. Somehow, in the busy day-to-day routine of family life, she had come to accept his challenges as normal and not something to worry about. Because her husband had similar bladder issues as a child, she adopted the attitude that Alex would simply outgrow the problem. As a family, health and fitness has not been a priority, and all of them are slightly overweight. Alex's upcoming camping trip may motivate his parents to seek medical help for his problems and to consider how their family might adopt a healthier lifestyle.

Most of us have an intellectual definition of health that we would use if someone asked us the question, "What does it mean to be healthy?" There is, however, often a wide discrepancy between what we believe and how we live our lives. We often make lifestyle choices that take us on paths that are contrary to what we say we want for our health and our lives. We may want to live long and healthy lives to enjoy our grandchildren, yet we don't heed the doctor's advice to lose some weight and get our diabetes under better control. While we may know what we should do, we all have places in our life where we make different choices. In the midst of our busy lives and many obligations, we may settle for a level of health that is tolerable rather than our ideal. The same holds true for our children. If our kids have runny noses all the time, we might simply blame it on bugs they catch at school and may not look more closely at what may be the problem. It may, in fact, be that we settle for fast food more nights than we had planned to or that we resort to more convenience foods at home than we had originally imagined when our children were infants.

It is helpful to clarify what you believe to be true about the health you want for yourself and your family and how you view your current health. Below are some questions to help you pay attention to these beliefs. Be sure to use an expanded definition of health that includes physical, emotional, social, and spiritual health rather than simply focusing on physical symptoms. Depression, loneliness, or feelings of hopelessness are also measures of your health.

Questions:

How would you describe your current state of health?

How would you describe the current state of health of your children?

Describe what your optimal level of health would look like and how your life would be different than it currently is if you achieved it.

Describe the optimal level of health you would like to achieve for your children. How would your children's lives be different if they achieved it?

If your child is old enough, ask them how they view their current state of health.

If your child identifies their health as less than optimal, ask them how they would like to feel?

If there is a discrepancy between your idea of the optimal health you would like to have and your current state of health, what do you think the reason is?

What symptoms are you or your children tolerating that are having a negative impact on your lives? What is preventing you from addressing these issues?

What concrete changes could you make in your life to improve the health challenges you or your children are facing?

On a scale of 1-10, how motivated are you to make these changes? If your motivation is lower than an 8, what could you do to increase your motivation? (We rarely make successful changes in our life unless we are highly motivated to do so.)

What health-related symptoms do you hope to improve by addressing the food sensitivities of your child? How will this impact their overall health? What will be the impact on his or her day-to-day life and future potential?

THE AMOUNT OF STRESS IN YOUR LIFE

Real-Life Story

> Ken's life can only be described as frantic. He is a single dad trying to balance his busy law practice while caring for his two school-aged children. When his wife died two years ago, he knew things would be difficult but was not prepared for all the challenges that have appeared. He hired a nanny to help during the day, but he still seems to come home at 7:00 p.m. to a sink full of dishes, homework still to be done, laundry piled in the hallway, and children mindlessly watching TV. His children's school performance has been sliding since his wife's death, but he never seems to get home in time to talk to the teachers. As well, the occasional tummy aches and runny noses they had as toddlers have become an almost daily occurrence and he rarely makes it through the week without a number of calls from the school saying one of his kids is sick and needs to go home.
>
> Ken is doing his best to keep his family afloat but feels like the ship is sinking. Even his own health is beginning to suffer, and he often has a severe headache by the end of his day. He has noticed that it takes at least five cups of coffee to keep him awake and alert so he can juggle the many demands of his life. He knows he needs to make some changes but can't even figure out where to begin.

The stress that Ken is experiencing in his life is causing so much distress that he is struggling to find a way to address the issues required to improve his own health and the health of his children. The death of his wife added many new challenges, as well as many additional things onto his already overflowing "to do" list. His children also appear to be suffering from the additional stress at home, as their school performance is deteriorating, and their physical symptoms seem to be increasing. When the stress level in a home is high, everyone is impacted. Attempting to change the diet of a family such as Ken's would be more than they all could cope with, and it would be recipe for failure. Something must be done to address the practical challenges in their home and decrease everyone's stress level before a diet change should be attempted.

Stress has a significant impact on all of us. The busy pace of your life and the many demands on your energy and time may be making it a challenge to find the rest and peace that your body, mind, and soul crave. Because you are reading this book, it is likely that you are experiencing physical and behavioral symptoms in your family that are escalating the stress and the worry in your home.

In times of stress, your body mobilizes many different mechanisms and resources to enable you to cope. With the release of adrenalin, your body gets ready to fight or flee. Your muscles tense, your mind gets clear, and your digestion shuts down as you are poised and ready to run. This adaption is useful for immediate, acute stress and enables you to mobilize all the resources you need to protect yourself. Unfortunately, much of the stress of your life is not acute and short-lived but chronic, persistent, and often overwhelming. Your body tries its best to cope, but week after week and month after month of this kind of heightened anxiety takes its toll. Eventually, your body gives up and gives in to the stress. Physical, behavioral, and psychological symptoms begin to appear, and your life begins to show the impact of this accumulated stress. You begin to develop back and neck pain, you seem to lose your keys every morning, and your energy level is so low that you seem to be dragging yourself through your day.

Food sensitivity symptoms in members of a family often increase the stress experienced by everyone. Whenever physical health deteriorates, the person will feel unwell and increasingly stressed by the symptoms. The longer they persist and the more they impact their life, the more difficult it will be to cope. If these symptoms result in a loss of your job or your child having frequent trips to the emergency department, your life may become overwhelmed by the challenge.

If the food sensitivity symptoms in yourself or your child are behavioral in nature, you may also be struggling to find the balance between discipline and affection for your child. Your daughter may be out of control, raging with tantrums, and so slow in doing things it is driving you crazy, or your son may be having so much trouble in school you feel like his second teacher. When you add this challenge to an already busy life, it is easy to see why stress is the result.

In addition, some of the neurological symptoms of food sensitivities increase feelings of frustration and anger—which, in turn, increases stress. Learning challenges, forgetfulness, irritability, tantrums, and a general difficulty in coping with the daily challenges of life may actually be the symptoms produced by the poorly tolerated food. Stress also increases many of the symptoms arising from the food that you are sensitive to. The good news here is that removal of the food produces a dramatic decrease in the levels of stress and the feeling of being overwhelmed. Whether the food is contributing to the stress or the stress is exacerbating the symptoms of the food, dealing with both of these issues can produce a significant change in the attitudes and feelings of calm in you and your children.

As you begin to adjust the diet of your family with the anticipation of finding better health, it is crucial that you look for ways to lower your stress level. If your life is like a runaway train where you are reacting rather than making conscious choices, it will be very difficult to add the additional time and energy that is required to be successful when you change your family's diet.

Below is a list of some of the physical, psychological, and behavioral symptoms of stress. Many of these symptoms are so common to us all that we minimize or ignore their impact. We push through our life and pay little or no attention to how we are feeling. The long-term cost on your health and quality of life is significant. If you do not address the issues early, your symptoms may increase and result in challenging physical, emotional, or behavioral problems. Whether stress is one of the contributing factors to the food sensitivity or whether the food sensitivity is one of the causes of the stress isn't as important as taking steps to improve the situation. Taking a positive step toward the resolution of any problem always lowers stress.

Symptoms of stress

Physical symptoms:

1. Headaches
2. Indigestion
3. Nausea
4. Vomiting
5. Palpitations
6. Difficulty taking a deep breath
7. Difficulty swallowing
8. Tingling in fingers or toes
9. Fatigue
10. Generalized aches and pains
11. Muscle twitches
12. Sweating
13. Muscle tension
14. Weight gain or weight loss
15. Shaking
16. Dry mouth
17. Insomnia
18. Poor balance
19. Lightheadedness or dizziness
20. Hyperventilation
21. Impairment of concentration
22. Impairment of memory
23. Coughing
24. Shortness of breath
25. Asthma symptoms when upset
26. Excessive yawning
27. Chest pain without any history of cardiac disease
28. Intestinal cramps

29. Diarrhea
30. Constipation
31. Urinary frequency
32. Uterine cramps
33. Decreased libido or sexual dysfunction
34. Frightening dreams
35. Elevated blood pressure
36. Low back pain

Psychological Symptoms:

1. Anxiety
2. Worry
3. Depression
4. Panic attacks
5. Negative outlook
6. Hopelessness
7. Fearfulness
8. Gloomy thoughts
9. Withdrawal
10. Feelings of unreality
11. Feeling unable to cope
12. Numbness or disconnection from feelings
13. Low frustration level
14. Crying
15. Feelings of sadness
16. Impaired problem-solving skills

Behavioral Symptoms:

1. Restlessness
2. Agitation
3. Making mistakes
4. Forgetfulness
5. Poor concentration
6. Violent outbursts

7. Change in usual behavior
8. Pacing
9. Hang-wringing
10. Indecision
11. Anger
12. Shouting
13. Irritability
14. Aggression
15. Eating too much or too little
16. Feeling unable to cope
17. Substance abuse (including alcohol)
18. Decreased motivation to participate in the normal activities of life
19. Procrastination

Questions:

What symptoms of stress from this list apply to you?

What symptoms have you been avoiding or not addressing in your own life? What has been preventing you from doing it?

What one action could you take today to lower your stress level with the intent of improving these symptoms?

As you look at the life of your child, what symptoms do you recognize in them that may be related to stress in their life?

What have you already tried in an effort to minimize these symptoms for your child? If your child is old enough, what have they done to help themselves?

What one action could you take today to lower the stress level of your child in an effort to improve these symptoms?

How might the stress level of your family decrease once the health, behavior, or learning-related symptoms of your child improve?

YOUR PAST EXPERIENCES WITH CHANGE

Real-Life Story

> Daphne has a newborn baby boy, Stephen, and a three-year-old daughter, Meghan. She has been a single mom for the last three months; her husband had an affair with a colleague and left unexpectedly. She is currently living at her parents' home in a new city. The changes in her life have felt like a whirlwind, and Daphne feels completely disoriented. Her daughter, Meghan, loves her grandparents but still asks daily, "When is Daddy coming home?"
>
> Daphne's new son, Stephen, has cried from the minute he was born and is causing a huge disruption in her parents' home. He seems inconsolable, no matter how long people walk him or cuddle him. Daphne is considering giving up breastfeeding in the hope that it will make things easier. The public health nurse made her weekly trip to check on Daphne and Stephen and suggested that Daphne consider staying off dairy products before she gives up breastfeeding to see if Stephen might settle down. Daphne simply rolled her eyes is despair and said plainly, "I can't take on one more change." The public health nurse reached over and touched Daphne's hand in a gentle gesture to ensure her that she understood. She remembered her days as a new mom struggling to make good decisions for her family but often feeling confused about what to do.
>
> Daphne has found herself in a place of change that she was unprepared for. The public health nurse helps her to recall places in her past where she has successfully navigated other changes and her anxiety begins to diminish. By recalling the resilience

she demonstrated in those situations, she is better able to find the courage to deal with her current challenges.

Daphne's past experiences with change can offer both support and discouragement, depending on the previous outcome of her effort. If she has attempted to change a situation many times in her life and has been unsuccessful, it may be a challenge to consider once again trying something new. The best way to overcome this hurdle is to help Daphne find something that matters significantly to her and to then use this as a motivator to change.

Readiness to Change

Changes happen often in life—whether by our own design or by being thrust upon us by some unsuspected circumstance. In chapter four, there is information both on what causes our resistance and the various stages of change. Our willingness to change a behavior—even if we know it is in our own best interest—varies significantly, depending on the issue. While we may be highly motivated to make some changes because the anticipated results are of great value to us, other changes create resistance, because we anticipate having to give up things we enjoy. If you feel it would be helpful, reread the section in chapter four on the stages of change and notice which one best describes how you are feeling now. Remember that you will move forward and back through these stages depending on a wide variety of circumstances.

As you consider the idea of changing the diet of your family, remember too that it is possible that you and your child may be at different stages of change. While you may be able to see the severity of your child's symptoms and the need for change, your child may think he or she is just fine and not see any reason to cooperate with the adjustments you want to make in their diet. Encouraging your child's cooperation requires careful consideration and planning—otherwise, they will likely sabotage your efforts often, and it will be difficult to know if the diet is making any difference at all. You will need to include them in conversation about the alternative foods you buy and help them to identify some motivating reason why they should give it a try for a month. You may even need to offer some type of reward or incentive to help them embrace the changes you are hoping to make.

Past Experiences with Change

There are many areas in your life where you have created successful habits—habits that truly support what you want your life to feel like. There have been times in your past where you have successfully made significant changes in order to get something that you really wanted. These past experiences will give important information as you begin the journey of changing the diet of your family. On the other hand, there may be other areas where you have attempted to make a change but feel that you have been unsuccessful. Below are two lists that give some ideas of things that support change and things that make it more difficult. Take a few minutes to read these lists before answering the questions that follow. Perhaps this will help you determine what might have made previous changes difficult and what you might do differently in this current situation to increase your chance of success.

Things That Make Change Easier

1. Someone who is willing to offer consistent support without judgment
2. Someone who is willing to listen with empathy when you talk about the changes you want to make
3. An increased desire to change because you are uncomfortable where you are
4. A naturally occurring transition in your life where you are forced to change for some external reason
5. Tools and information to help you know how to actually make the change
6. An understanding of the values that you are honoring more fully by making the change
7. An understanding of the needs that have been driving your previous behavior

116

8. Connection with other people who are facing similar challenges or who are trying to make similar changes
9. Changing things in your physical environment to allow things to *feel* different, thereby supporting other kinds of changes
10. Sharing your plans with someone who is supportive and will hold you accountable
11. Substituting another enjoyable behavior for the one you are changing
12. Rewarding yourself for your successes
13. Setting realistic expectations and planning small steps
14. Making only one change at a time
15. Financial resources that support the changes you want to make
16. A work and personal schedule and pace of life that allows time to make the change
17. An ability to see places in your past where you have made successful changes

Things That Make Change Difficult

1. Criticism and doubt from other people in your life
2. Too many demands from others
3. Too many things on your "to do" list imposed by others
4. Too many things on your "to do" list that you put there yourself
5. Financial pressure
6. Pressure from extended family members, such as parents and grandparents
7. Longstanding habits that are difficult to break
8. Stories from your past that create self-doubt
9. Work pressures that take up excess time or create excess stress
10. Fear of change
11. Lack of readiness to change
12. Not enough support for the change

13. Preferring immediate gratification rather than patiently waiting for sustainable change
14. Attempting a large change without taking small, manageable steps first
15. Lack of understanding and awareness of what has driven your past, inappropriate choices
16. Lack of support and people willing to hold you accountable for the changes you want to make
17. Lack of knowledge or tools to facilitate a successful change
18. A sense of denial and an inability to recognize the need for change

Questions:

Identify a change in your life you have successfully made or a positive habit you successfully developed?

What personal strengths and qualities did you draw on to be successful?

What motivated you to want to change?

What support did you have then that made it easier to be successful?

What influences can you identify in your own life that has made change easier? (Refer to the previous list on things that make change easier if you need some ideas.)

What influences can you identify that make change more difficult for you? (Refer to the previous list on things that make change more difficult if you need some ideas.)

As you look at your child's strengths, which ones will support him or her to embrace and be motivated to make the changes you are asking?

What influences in your child's life will support their ability to make these changes?

What influences in your child's life will impede their ability to make these changes?

What is the first, concrete step you can take that will support the change you want to make in the diet of your child?

THE CONNECTION OF YOUR MOTIVATION TO SOMETHING YOU VALUE

Real-Life Story

Chelsea and Robert live with their three children in the basement suite of Chelsea's parents' home. Robert is a student finishing his medical degree, and Chelsea is committed to staying home to care for their three young children. They were reluctant at first to accept Chelsea's parents' offer to live with them but knew that while Robert made enough for them to live on, he didn't make enough for them to afford an apartment or house big enough for their growing family. Chelsea's parents had welcomed their daughter and her family and were excited at the idea of having their grandchildren close. They knew the family would be moving soon, as Robert would begin a medical practice in a new city the following year, so everyone was committed to making the living arrangement work.

Chelsea and Robert want to be independent, so Chelsea is clear with her mother that she will be making meals for her own family and organizing their weekly activities. While she loves Sunday dinners upstairs with her folks, she loves caring for her own family the rest of the time. Chelsea's kids enjoy regular fun time and even sleepovers with their nana and granddad, but Chelsea is very careful to honor her parents' need for privacy, as well. When some friction arose because Chelsea's parents were not consistently honoring the children's special diet needs, Chelsea, Robert and her parents sat down over a cup of tea in the evening to find solutions rather than allow any animosities to build. Chelsea and Robert want their children to be healthy and active, and they know that keeping them off apple juice, dairy products and junk food makes a significant difference in their behavior as well as their health. They are hopeful their parents will understand. Both families value their relationship with one another so highly that they are committed to talking openly and honestly with each other and are usually able to find workable solutions.

In order to honor the high value Chelsea and Robert place on family connection and health, they try to look for solutions that respect everyone's point of view. Even when small challenges appear, they are highly motivated to make the situation work because they want their children to be nurtured in an environment that fosters their sense of belonging. They stand behind what they believe is right for their children and are able to enlist the support and cooperation of Chelsea's parents through calm conversation.

The best motivation to make a positive change comes from within. You change because you can see the value of the change and trust that it will make a difference in your life in some meaningful way. The choice honors what you want and what you value most. The interesting thing about values is that they are unique to each of us and don't fluctuate very much over our lifetimes. Most of the things that are important to you now were an important part of your life as a child. Even as your life circumstances change, values usually remain constant. Honoring them is the path to a fulfilling life. The power of getting clear on what you value and then using this as a road map for decision-making is amazing. I often have my clients carry their values list in their purse or wallet so they can refer to it when they find themselves in places of indecision.

Clarification of Values

If you were able to make choices based entirely on what you value most, how would you change what you are currently doing? Below is a list of common values. At the end of the accompanying questions, there will be a place where you can write down your final list of the values that matter most to you. You can then use these to support your motivation to change your family's diet.[27.]

Questions:

As you read the list below, mark the words that jump out at you. Some of these values will be so important that they influence the direction of your life. Feel free to combine similar words or to add words that are not on the list. Choose ten of them and write them in the spaces that follow the remaining questions. If your child is old enough, please consider doing this exercise with them as well. It is very helpful for them to understand what supports healthy choices and what will motivate them to choose wisely. The information will also help support your child to be motivated enough to cooperate with diet changes you are making as well as other aspects of your life.

Value Words

Accomplishment	Excellence	Orderliness
Accuracy	Faith	Participation
Achievement	Family	Partnership
Acknowledgement	Focus	Peace
Adventure	Free Spirit	Performance
Aesthetics	Freedom	Personal growth
Altruism	Fun	Power
Authenticity	Growth	Privacy
Autonomy	Harmony	Recognition
Balance	Health	Resilience
Beauty	Honesty	Results
Bonding	Humor	Risk taking

Certainty	Independence	Romance
Clarity	Integrity	Security
Collaboration	Intimacy	Self expression
Commitment	Joy	Sensuality
Comradeship	Leadership	Service
Connection	Learning	Solitude
Contribution	Love	Spirituality
Creativity	Loyalty	Success
Determination	Magic	To be heard
Directness	Mastery	Tradition
Elegance	Moderation	Trust
Emotional health	Nature	Truthfulness
Empowerment	Nurture	Vitality
Environment	Openness	Zest

Your own ideas below

1.   2.   3.

Questions:

Now take some time to reflect on the following questions. You may need to refer on the list above for ideas.

Close your eyes and imagine a time in your life when you felt totally at peace and happy. What were you doing? Where were you, and who was with you? What is important to you about this situation? Notice what you are experiencing. What sights and sounds did you notice? Look at what you have written and identify what important values are contained in your story.

Take a minute to imagine that you are about five years old and are playing in your favorite place, doing your favorite thing. Close your eyes and really connect to the experience. Imagine the sights, sounds, smells, textures, and emotion of the experience. What are you doing? Who are you with? What feelings do you notice? Take a few minutes to jot down your story; then take a minute to identify any values that are evident in your story.

If someone were writing a speech to honor you, what would you most like them to say? What does that tell you about what is important to you?

Listing your values

From the previous exercises, write down a list of the values you have identified as being most important in your life.

VALUES AS YOU IDENTIFIED THEM FROM THE PREVIOUS QUESTIONS

1.
2.
3.
4.
5.
6.
7.
8.
9.
10.

Now take a few minutes to rank the list of values you have created in the order that reflects how you are living them in your life today, and list them below.

VALUES RANKED AS YOU ARE LIVING THEM TODAY

1.
2.
3.
4.
5.

6.

7.

8.

9.

10.

Now take a few minutes to rank the list of values you have created in the order that reflects how you would like them to be represented in your ideal life. This exercise will help you identify the high-priority items that you want to spend your time on and help you notice where your priorities are currently out of balance. Internal motivation will be the highest when you are working toward something that appears at the top of your ideal values list. If you are spending countless hours on something that is actually a low priority for you, it is an energy drain and should be removed from your calendar to allow space and energy for the things that really matter.

VALUES RANKED AS YOU WOULD LIVE THEM IN YOUR IDEAL LIFE

1.

2.

3.

4.

5.

6.

7.

8.

9.

10.

What have you learned from doing this exercise?

If there is a discrepancy between how you are living your values today and the way you would like them to be, take a minute to write down what you think is getting in the way.

What action could you take today to begin to move these two lists more in line with each other?

Take time to consider how the values you have identified will support successful diet change. For example, if one of your highest values was family, notice how your love and commitment to them will help you manage adversity and frustration when they appear.

What physical object or reminder could you create to help you stay committed to the values that are supporting your desire to change the diet of your family? For example, placing a picture of your family on your refrigerator may be a reminder of why you are taking such extra care in your cooking.

THE BALANCE OF YOUR BUSY LIFE

Real-Life Story

Carolyn and David have been married for eight years and have very busy lives. Their son, Evan, who has recently been diagnosed with ADHD, is the only child they have had together. David has two daughters, age fourteen and twelve, who live with them on the weekends, and Carolyn has a daughter, aged eleven, who lives with them full-time. Carolyn and David are both committed to creating a balanced life for their family but are discovering it is far more difficult than they had imagined. Evan has multiple medical and counseling appointments every month, and each of the older girls has extensive athletic and music commitments. By the time the family calendar for the week is created, there isn't any space at all for Carolyn and David to spend time together except late in the evening, when they are both exhausted. The dietician has suggested they try a dairy-free, additive-free diet for Evan to see if it might improve his symptoms and decrease his need for Ritalin, which the school is pressuring them to try. They are feeling swamped and overwhelmed at the idea of adding one more thing to their already busy lives.

Before taking on this additional challenge, Carolyn and David decide to seek the support of a life coach. They are aware that if they don't make some significant changes and establish clearer priorities, the family stress level will continue to rise. With the support of their coach, Carolyn and David have been able to make adjustments in their lives that allowed them to set clearer boundaries between work and family life and to establish a family calendar that honors their desire for a peace and balance in their home. Once they let go of the areas in their life that had been draining their energy, they were able to find the time and support to begin adjusting Evan's diet. Carolyn and David are committed to offering each of their children the best opportunity possible to reach their potential and they now feel better able to achieve this goal.

In order to make space in your life for the additional work created by adjustments in diet, it is important to ensure there is room. Simply adding another job to an already-runaway life is a recipe for failure before you begin. Even if you are clear about what you want your life to be like, it is often difficult to make the appropriate choices because of all the different demands placed on you. How do you actually go about slowing your life down? How do you find time for the things that matter in the midst of the requests that everyone else has of you?

It can very helpful to put all the pieces of your life on a page in front of you and take a thoughtful look at them. Doing this begins a process of intentionally choosing what you make time for in your life and what you are doing that you wish you could let go of.

Below, there is a diagram entitled the Wheel of Life.[28.] It is a circle that resembles a pie and is divided into eight different sections. Underneath the diagram is a list of words that represent various parts of your life. Read the words and decide which ones best identify the areas that comprise the different aspects of your life. There are many possibilities, so choose your own words if you don't see ones on the list that fit. Take the words and place each of them in one of the sections of the diagram. If you have chosen more than eight words, divide some of the sections in half.

Once you have placed the words on the circle, take a few minutes to write down how satisfied you are with each section of your life. For example, if you love to exercise but have been unable to find the time to be active, you might decide that the area marked as fitness on your circle my rank only a two out of ten. On the other hand, if your relationship with your husband is amazing, you might score that one as nine out of ten. Be sure when you are deciding on a number that you are evaluating how happy you are with this part of your life. Do not fall into the trap of ranking them based on the opinions or judgments of someone else.

It is important to notice that the lines between the sections are dotted. This is done in order to emphasize the fact that the areas of your life are intimately connected. For example, if you decide to increase the amount of space in your week for exercise, it may increase your energy, improve your relationships with your family, allow you to make some new friendships, and significantly improve your health. This is an important thing to consider, as one small change in your schedule can have a big impact on your life.

WHEEL OF LIFE

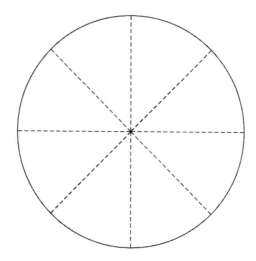

Independence	Personal growth
Family	Friends
Significant other/romance	Career
Physical environment	Faith
Rest and solitude	Health
Finances	Support
Contribution	Creativity
Fun and recreation	Freedom to make your own choices

Questions:

Once you have completed this, take a look at all the sections and notice which section is calling for some type of attention first? Which one needs to be adjusted or managed in order for you to make room for the extra time to adjust your family's diet? Is the lowest one draining your energy? Do you need more of the highest one? Is one of them mediocre but actually impacting all the others? Make a thoughtful and intentional choice.

What area of your life do you feel is most in need of support or change?

Brainstorm some ideas for how to manage this area of your life. Don't judge your answers. Simply be creative in your thoughts and jot down anything at all that comes to mind.

1.
2.
3.
4.
5.
6.
7.
8.

From the previous section on values, take out the page where you prepared the list of values as you would like to live them in your ideal life. Place the list of the ideas you have just brainstormed next to the list of your values and notice which ideas are most in line with what is important to you. If you have to, create a totally new solution that is based more closely on your values. For example, if one of your ideas to address your lack of exercise is to go for a walk early in the morning before your kids get up and you place a high value on peace and solitude, this choice has an increased chance of working better than a decision to go to a noisy, crowded gym.

What action(s) will you take that will allow you more time to address the diet of your family while honoring something that you value highly in your life?

How will this make the additional work of changing the diet of your family easier and more fun?

What will motivate you to make these changes in your life today?

What things that are draining your time and your energy will you remove from your life? These will often be things you are doing for someone else rather than things that are honoring your own values.

What ripple effect can you see that will result from your changes that may address other issues and challenges in your life?

If your child is old enough, please complete the questions in this section with them. Helping them to be intentional about the choices and priorities of their life will help them cope more easily with the diet changes and also teach them great skills they can use for the rest of their life.

THE IMPACT OF YOUR OLD STORIES AND BELIEFS

Real-Life Story

As she walks across the stage at her graduation as a nurse, Tara is proud of her perseverance. When she became pregnant at seventeen, just before graduating from high school, Tara believed her dream of becoming a pediatric nurse was forever lost. She left high school to care for her new son, Matthew, and lived at home with her parents. Many of her friends left her small hometown and went on to university many miles away. Tara kept herself busy caring for Matthew and working at the local grocery store to make ends meet while taking courses in the evening to finish high school.

Matthew was a difficult child—even as an infant—and seemed to have one health problem after another. He had constant colds, was underweight for his age and by the age of three he already had had two bouts of pneumonia. Tara spent many hours in doctors' offices and searching the Internet for answers to Matthew's health challenges. Finally, she discovered a website that addressed the topic of food sensitivities and began to read stories similar to her son's.

With the support of her parents, Tara found a doctor in the next town who was an expert in food sensitivities in children and made an appointment for Matthew. The doctor confirmed what Tara had suspected, and her son was placed on a one-month diet that removed the two most common foods he ate and the ones she loves, as well—eggs and bananas.

After being on the diet for only a week, Matthew's symptoms disappeared quickly, and he began to gain weight and grow taller. Tara was so inspired by the transformation in Matthew's health that she began to dream again of being a nurse who worked with children. Perhaps she could help educate other families about the power of changing the diets of their children. Despite her fear of not being smart enough to succeed, and her belief when she left high school as a single mom that she would never be able to continue her education, Tara enrolled in nursing school.

Many of her classmates were much younger, and Tara often felt alone. After a few months, however, she put these concerns behind her, and began to excel in her studies. The wisdom and life experience she had gained caring for Matthew gave her real-life experience to draw from. As she now walks across the stage to the sound of applause from both her parents and Matthew, Tara smiles and is proud of her perseverance. Her old fears of not being smart and the stigma of being a single mom who dropped out of high school are behind her. She has made her dream come true after all.

Tara's story illustrates the impact that the experiences of our past can have on our current choices. When Tara left high school to have a baby, she felt the criticism and judgment of her peers and other adults in her life. As she courageously made choices based on what was important to her, her confidence increased, and she began to believe that she could achieve her dream of being a nurse, despite her difficult start. The old stories from her past were left behind.

We all have old tapes that play in our heads and impact how we think of ourselves. The adults in our lives—no matter how caring they are—still say and do things that impact our beliefs about ourselves. This, in turn, has a significant impact on what we do and why we do it. For example, a child growing up might be told that he is not a particularly good athlete and consistently be encouraged to choose other activities. When he reaches adulthood, he longs for better health and fitness and dreams of training for a marathon, but quickly dismisses the idea because his old tape tells him he won't be able to do it. Unless we increase our awareness of these old stories and tapes, we continue to use them to make our decisions as adults.

The flip side of old stories, however, is that they may also offer support. Another adult who was reminded often what an amazing athlete she was as a child will find it much easier to make a choice to train for a marathon as an adult. Her old story actually supports her life decisions rather than impeding them.

Pema Chodrun, an author and Buddhist nun, describes three reactions we all use to respond to these triggers from our past in her book *Taking the Leap—Freeing Ourselves from Old Habits and Fears*. We might numb them over completely and simply be unaware of their impact in our lives. We might turn to addictions of many types, such as food, work, alcohol, drugs, sex, or exercise. We also can resort to blame and negativity, where we respond in anger to the people in our lives or turn that anger inward and develop self-judgment that becomes paralyzing in our lives. Our main desire, whichever strategy we use, is to get away from the discomfort we are feeling. Pema uses a wonderful analogy to make this point by comparing what we are feeling to a child suffering from poison ivy. "Because we want to relieve the discomfort, we automatically scratch and it seems a perfectly sane thing to do. In the face of anything we don't like, we automatically try to escape. In other words, scratching is our habitual way of trying to get away, trying to escape our fundamental discomfort, the fundamental itch of restlessness and insecurity, or that very uneasy feeling that something bad is about to happen."[43]

By increasing our awareness of these old stories and finding the courage to step past the shame and fear they may offer, their power over our lives begins to diminish. Rather that resort to our default, inappropriate coping strategies, we can choose to simply acknowledge the discomfort we are feeling. We can stop itching furiously and making our experience worse and, instead, seek wise counsel from someone we trust to find a different answer. We must allow ourselves to feel the experiences of our lives rather than find ways to avoid them in order to grow. By embracing the old stories that strengthen our courage and resilience and increase our willingness to change, we can increase the likelihood that we will make more empowering choices.

Questions:

What words would you use to describe the weaknesses you believe you have? After you make the list, take a minute to notice if they are actually true or if they are words that someone else has labeled you with.

What words would you use to describe your strengths? After you make the list, take a minute to notice where in life you were encouraged to develop these strengths.

What labels and beliefs from your past do you think will make it difficult for you to remove the trigger food from the diet of your family? (For example, your mother might have told you that you weren't a good cook, or your dad may have often referred to you as lazy and unmotivated.)

What labels and beliefs from your past do you think will support you being successful in removing the trigger food from the diet of your family? (For example, your hockey coach may have commented on your tenacious perseverance, or your mom may have reinforced your healthy and nutritious food choices.)

If your child is old enough, consider helping them to also answer these questions. Often even very young children have developed ideas about who they are based on feedback they have already been given. It is a great exercise to help them identify the strengths that they have and learn to acknowledge the areas where they might want to grow a little.

YOUR ABILITY TO SET HEALTHY BOUNDARIES

Real-Life Story

Debbie and Raymond have one-year-old twins, Charlotte and Ashley, who keep them busy juggling all the demands in their lives. Raymond works as a salesman and is often out of town, and Debbie works part-time as an accountant. The three days a week that Debbie works, Raymond's mother looks after their daughters. Because both girls were born prematurely and were hospitalized for the first month of their lives, it is difficult to get them into any type of routine. They each nap and want to eat at different times. Caring for them is a full-time job. Debbie continues to breastfeed the girls, as she has been encouraged to do so by the doctor in order to help their immune systems develop and decrease the girls' chances of developing food sensitivities.

While Debbie and Raymond are very grateful to Raymond's mom for helping them while Debbie works, they are very frustrated by her lack of support in following their wishes for the girls' care. She is convinced that Debbie has breastfed them long enough and often tries to sneak in a bottle of formula rather than breast milk during the day to show their parents they would do fine. While Debbie and Raymond know that caring for their children is a lot of work, they are clear that they want their daughters to eat the food that will help prevent them having food sensitivities in later years.

Debbie and Raymond are now trying to decide how to convey their wishes and priorities to Raymond's parents without creating a confrontation. They have been doing some reading from a book on boundaries and are committed to finding a strategy to express their concerns in a clear yet compassionate way. They are also aware, however, that they may need to consider alternate daycare

> arrangements for their girls if Raymond's mom will not hear their
> concerns.

One of the biggest challenges for all of us (and the topic of many parenting books) is the issue of boundaries. Boundaries are the imaginary lines that we draw around ourselves that allow us to claim the places where we choose what is right for us. We all have places where we will let others come close, and we all have places where we keep people at a distance. Henry Cloud and John Townsend have written a number of successful books on the topic of boundaries and have even written one entitled *Safe People*. This book encourages us all to create a circle of caring people in our lives and to successfully identify how we would know who these people might be. Just as we teach our small children to avoid strangers and to honor the feelings they have related to inappropriate touching, so we as adults need to be very clear where our personal boundaries are. When is someone's request of us too much, given our already busy lives? When are the demands of our bosses too far outside our job description for what we are able to manage? When are the obligations of caring for aging parents outside of what we can do?

This issue of boundaries is an important one as you embark on a plan to change your family's diet. There will be no shortage of people telling you how foolish they think you are and offering you their unsolicited advice. They may try to influence your children and convince both of you that "just a little won't hurt!" You will need to clarify what you want for yourself and your family. You may have to frequently remind people that the health of your family is your responsibility and that you are very capable of doing the job on your own. Some of your boundaries are connected to old stories. Sometimes you will give in to people simply because you have always been taught to be nice and helpful to others. You may have trouble speaking up for what you want and instead let others decide for you.

Learning to stand up for what you value, what you need, and what will make your life the life you are longing for is an essential skill for us all to learn. First, you must clarify what you want, as you did with your wheel of life and values exercises. It is then helpful to get clear on the choices you are prepared to make and then to set appropriate boundaries to protect what you want from the unwelcome influence of others.

It is also important, however, to be aware of the impact that *your* choices have on others. Again, old stories can appear, and you may find yourself crossing over the boundaries of others to get what you want for yourself. Honoring boundaries works both ways.

One of the most helpful and empowering pieces of learning that children get from adjusting to diet changes is the ability to stand up for what is right for them. They learn early to say no when inappropriate foods are offered and can become very savvy at an early age in asking for what they want. This strengthens their ability to say no to drugs, alcohol, sex, and other inappropriate activities arising from peer pressure.

Questions:

Learning how to set healthy boundaries is an important skill for your child. If your child is old enough, please consider helping them to answer the following questions. Connecting to places in their life where they successfully set a firm boundary and places where they felt intimidated and not able to speak up will help them problem solve how they will deal with situations that arise related to the changes in diet.

Describe a situation where you honored your boundaries and stood up for something you needed or wanted. How did you feel in this situation?

Describe a situation where someone stepped over your boundaries and you had to respond to what had happened. What did you do? How did you feel?

Imagine a situation where boundary challenges might arise with respect to the alteration of your family's diet, and brainstorm how you will handle it. Remember to connect to the value-based reasons for making the decision to address the needs of your child and your family.

YOUR ABILITY TO MOVE PAST YOUR OWN DOUBTS AND SABOTEURING VOICES

Real-Life Story

> Karen has decided that today will be the day she will take control of her diet. Today will be the day she will stick to the plan the dietician has created for her.
>
> The day began well as she ate her piece of fruit, bowl of bran cereal with skim milk, and soft-boiled egg before heading off to work. She packed her lunch with only a salad and a piece of fruit and decided to treat herself to a latte to go with it. After all, this counted as only a beverage and a dairy product. As the day continued and the stress at Karen's work increased, she could feel herself eyeing the donuts brought in by one of her coworkers. She knew they weren't on her plan, but she eventually gave in and decided to have just one. A little later on in the day, one became two, and she grabbed a third as she walked out the door to go home.
>
> Karen got home and looked in the mirror as she took off her coat. The little nagging voice that was so familiar to her began to chat again. It reminded her that she was "weak, lazy, and undisciplined" and "not even committed enough to her health to stay on the diet for one full day." She tossed her coat on the floor and headed to the fridge for a snack. *Who cares, anyway?* she thought. *I am fat, and that is too bad.*
>
> The voice in Karen's head is a familiar one that encourages her often to sabotage her efforts at self-discipline and stay committed to her health. Her mother had criticized her all through her childhood for not being strong enough to make better choices. She had frequently commented on her weight and regularly compared

> her to her very slim and athletic sister. Although her mother had passed away years ago, this voice continues to sabotage Karen's efforts to improve her own health.

We all have this troublesome, negative, sabotaging voice that chats away in our heads and tells us things like, "You aren't good enough," "You aren't smart enough," "You won't be able to do it," "People won't love you if you make them angry," or "You have to do things for others all the time in order to have friends." We all have our own special voices, and the words that are spoken are usually connected to some old stories in our lives.[29.] The persona of the saboteur may take on different forms, but the voices are often ones we recognize. Your voice might be a critical parent, a difficult teacher, an angry boss, or a nasty older brother. Often, the saboteur thinks he is protecting us and keeping us safe by doing everything possible to maintain the status quo, but he actually makes us live in fear and limitation. The saboteur hates change of any kind, and the closer the change gets, the louder his objections become. Because of his aversion to you becoming stronger and empowered, the saboteur loves it when you sell yourself out and allow others to walk all over your boundaries.

If the voice of your saboteur becomes loud and persistent, it convinces you that you are not worthy and you slink back from your lives in shame. As Brene Brown writes in her book, *I Thought It Was Just Me But It Wasn't,* shame resilience requires several things: (1) the ability to recognize and understand the triggers that connect us to old stories and the experience of shame; (2) high levels of critical awareness that allow us to make connections between our private lives and the social, political, and economic influences around us; (3) the willingness to reach out to others to share our experiences and have them heard by safe and empathetic people; and (4) the ability to speak about shame and not hide our feelings, believe these stories are true, or numb these experiences away.[42.]

One of the strategies for "Taming Your Saboteur" is to acknowledge its presence and create a physical image of what it looks like. By doing this, it is much easier to disconnect from the negative energy the saboteur's voice creates in your life. An example of this saboteur imagery might be a character named Ivy. Ivy resembles a plant that grows like a weed all over your body. She might cling so tightly that you are unable to move, exercise, help yourself, or even speak as she twists herself around your throat. She is very persistent in her desire to cling to you, and it requires major garden tools and great courage to break free. She clings particularly tightly when you decide to increase your fitness and reminds you that you aren't really an athlete at all. She also chokes back your words when you try to speak up for yourself and prefers you to simply be quiet and behave at the mercy of others. By connecting to this image and then actively speaking words to tell Ivy to go on an extended vacation in the garden, the energy of doubt she creates disappears almost immediately.

The voice of the saboteur is sure to appear whenever you make a mistake in a food you offer your child or when things don't work out perfectly, the way you had hoped. It will also be reinforced in the doubts and comments of many of the people in your life. The voice of the saboteur is often the reason that people abandon the process of diet change altogether and slide back into their old ways of eating. Their children's health, behavior, and learning are compromised, and their symptoms may continue to worsen.

Questions:

Take a few minutes to complete the following sentences and connect to the unique voice and appearance of your own saboteur. *If your child is old enough, please also play with this activity to help them identify the voice of doubt and criticism that appears in their own thoughts.*

THE PERSONA OF YOUR SABOTEUR

Hi, my name is

My appearance suits my personality. A good description of me would be

I am the kind of character who

I torture you by

I typically get you to think

I also make you feel

Which makes you do

My favorite time to influence your thoughts and your beliefs about yourself is when

You will know I am around when you notice

HOW TO MOVE PAST THE VOICE OF YOUR SABOTEUR

The main thought that your saboteur wants you to believe is

Is this thought really true about you?

How do you react when you believe this thought is true?

How would you react if you didn't believe it was true?

What do you actually know to be true about the story your saboteur is trying to tell you?

The things that silence your saboteur and make it difficult for it to influence you are

The circumstances in which your saboteur is most likely to appear when you change the diet of your family are

YOUR WILLINGNESS TO ASK FOR HELP

Real-Life Story

Gordon and Thelma live on their own, much to the dismay of their grown children. They are both eighty years old and are managing just fine, as far as they are concerned. No, they can't clean the house as well as they used to, but they certainly don't need a cleaning lady yet. They don't cook fancy meals anymore, but they have their groceries delivered and survive quite well on soup and sandwiches. When their kids suggested they move to a senior home, they dug in their heels and refused to go.

Gordon and Thelma's daughter, Frances, lives two blocks away from her parents and is exhausted caring for them. They are so forgetful that they often leave the stove on when they are finished cooking, and she is constantly afraid one of them will fall going up and down the steep stairs to their bedroom. She takes them dinner at least four nights a week and does her best to get them to their doctor's appointments. Her own family is struggling as she spreads herself so thin. She has two teenage sons at home who need her support, as both have ADHD and have multiple tutoring appointments during the week. Fran is also doing her best to give them a dairy-free, gluten-free diet. Her husband is wonderful but travels with his business and isn't always available to help. Fran's sister and brother live about an hour away from their parents and leave most of the care and day-to-day decisions to Fran.

Fran needs some help but is reluctant to ask for it. She has no idea where to go to find professional help for her parents; therefore, she gives in to their insistence to stay in their house. Fran finds it difficult to admit to her siblings that she is struggling for fear they will come and take her parents to live closer to them. Because she is the youngest sibling, she also wants to prove to them that she can do it in order to dispel their childhood label that she is spoiled and lazy. Fran is exhausted from caring for them, but she doesn't want to lose them, either. She feels trapped and alone.

Fran's story is an example of a mother caught in the sandwich generation between aging parents and growing children. Her reluctance to ask for support from her siblings is partially based on stories from her childhood. Her saboteur's voice quickly reminds her that asking for help indicates that she is spoiled and lazy. Instead of being courageous and standing up for herself, she allows her siblings to walk all over her boundaries. Because Fran wants to offer her boys the best support she can to deal with their ADHD, she pushes herself to keep to a schedule that leaves no time at all for her own priorities. Fran desperately needs to take a look at the obligations in her life and decide which ones are draining her energy and need to be let go. If she doesn't make some changes soon, it is very likely that Fran's health will also begin to deteriorate.

If you are to be successful in changing longstanding habits, finding safe places to go and ask for help is crucial. Going it alone in the belief that you should be able to do it that way will likely lead to recurrent failure. How do you ask for help in a way that will support you getting what you need? What obstacles get in the way of you asking for help? How would you recognize a safe person with whom to share your thoughts and ask for help?

Sharing your plans for change with someone else dramatically increases your likelihood of success. Once you have found a safe person to ask and are clear on what you need, take the risk and do it. Ask them to hold you accountable for the action you want to take and to check up on you to see that you stay on course. Notice the statistics below that are taken from the Coachville coaching website[30.] on successful change. The percentage values indicate the likelihood that you will make your anticipated change successfully. Accountability significantly increases your odds of success so find someone who cares enough to ask how you are doing.

- You hear an idea—10%
- Decide when you will do it—40%
- Plan how you will do it—50%
- Commit to someone else you will do it—65%
- Have a specific accountability deadline with the person you've committed to—95%

After reading some of the suggestions below, take a minute and answer the questions that follow. This will give you a picture of how easy or difficult it is for you to ask for help. Please also help your child identify areas where they may need to enlist the help of others and develop some strategies to make that easier to do.

Obstacles to Asking For Help

1. A disempowering belief that asking for help implies weakness
2. A lack of safe people to ask
3. A lack of safe people who are willing to step up and actually make time to help
4. A lack of clarity about the type of help that you need
5. Feelings of being so overwhelmed by your circumstance and your life that you can't recognize your need for help
6. A belief that no one else can do it as well as you can
7. A belief that doing a lot for others will get you the love and attention you crave so you spend excessive amounts of time helping others
8. A belief you have the answers for everyone else's life if only they would listen
9. People in your life who take over when you simply ask for a little support

Things That Facilitate Asking For Help

1. People willing to listen without telling you how to fix your situation
2. People who offer you their full attention (e.g., eye contact) when you are talking to them
3. People who are interested in your story and willing to ask curious questions rather than impose judgments

4. People who know you well enough that they can remind you of your past successes when you are caught up in a difficult situation
5. A belief that asking for help is a sign of courage and strength rather than weakness
6. A true desire to slow down the pace of your life and to find solutions that offer more balance
7. The willingness to take the time to look at your problem to try and determine what the need or old story is that is driving you rather than focusing on the small details
8. The willingness to allow the other people in your life to make their own choices and mistakes without needing to rescue them
9. Doing exercises such as the wheel of life to increase clarity on the balance of your life
10. The ability to recognize the voice of the saboteur when self-doubt appears and question what is really true
11. The willingness to let go of your perfectionism
12. A commitment to finding a way to ask for help without making it sound like a demand
13. Clarity about the type of help you need

Questions:

What obstacles do you face in your life that makes it difficult to ask for help when you need it?

What beliefs do you hold about asking for help? Do you consider asking for help to be a sign of strength or a sign of weakness?

What increases your willingness to ask for help when you need it?

Give an example of a time in your life when you asked for help and were successful in getting it.

Give an example of a time in your life when you didn't ask for help and now feel you should have. What prevented you from asking for help?

Who in your life offers you the experience of being able to ask for help without judgment, criticism, or a need to fix your situation?

As you step up to change the diet of your family, what support do you need? Where will you go to find it? What will increase your willingness to ask?

What accountability are you prepared to share with a safe person in your life who will support you to make the changes in diet and in your life that you want? While the word *deadline* may conjure up images of term papers and assignments, in this case, honoring this deadline will ultimately serve you and your family in life-changing ways.

YOUR WILLINGNESS TO ADDRESS ISSUES RELATED TO YOUR OWN HEALTH

Real-Life Story

Cari hopes she has finally found some answers to the serious health problems of her son, Daniel. Daniel, who is twelve years old, suffers from severe asthma and has been unable to participate in active sports for most of his life. This condition is particularly bothersome during the cold weather, so he is forced to spend many of his winter days indoors.

Cari attended a workshop on food sensitivities and became convinced that dairy products were Daniel's trigger foods as he ate them several times a day. He loves yogurt for breakfast and she can barely keep up with the amount of chocolate milk he drinks. She is hopeful that removing dairy products from Daniel's diet will make a difference and is trying to enlist the support of her husband, Oliver, for her idea.

She is unprepared for Oliver's response. He insisted on seeing multiple scientific studies to prove the theory and flatly refused to stop drinking the milk he loved. He had drunk milk all his life and couldn't see how it had had any negative impact on his health. When Cari attempted to share with him what she had learned at the workshop, he refused to listen. Yes, maybe he had gas now and then, and perhaps that eczema on his hands was embarrassing, and yes, he had struggled a lot in school as a child, but he doubted that these issues were related to anything he was eating.

After much discussion, Oliver agreed to support Cari's efforts to remove dairy products from Daniel's diet but has flatly refused to change what he eats. He insists on leaving the ice cream in the freezer and the milk in the fridge, even though it makes avoiding them more difficult for Daniel. Cari only hopes that if Daniel's health improves significantly, perhaps Oliver will change his mind and finally get some relief from his own health and learning challenges, as well.

As in the case of Oliver, one of the biggest obstacles that I see in parents considering a change in their children's diet is reluctance to remove the food from their own diet. In these situations it is common for one or both parents to over consume the same food they are trying to remove from their child's diet. Rather than face the fact that perhaps they, too, have many symptoms of food sensitivity, they prefer to minimize their own health challenges. The symptoms in children rarely occur in isolation and it is common for a number of family members to suffer from similar issues.

Questions:

As a parent, I ask you to consider the questions below and be honest with yourself about the state of your own health. If there are symptoms impacting your own life, be a role model for your child and embrace the changes along with them. There is great power in modeling successful change for your children and great potential for a significant improvement in your own health, as well as your child's.

Take another look at the list of food sensitivity symptoms in chapter one. What symptoms are you experiencing now or did you experience as a child?

What other health problems are you facing that are not on this list that you are avoiding getting treatment for?

What five foods would you identify as the ones that you love and eat most often?

What food is the one that you would find most difficult to give up?

When I asked you to complete the questionnaire about your child in chapter three, were you hesitant to identify this food because removing it from your family's diet felt difficult for you? Why do you think that was?

What similarities do you see between your child's symptoms and your own—either now or in the past?

What similarities do you see between the foods your child craves and the ones you love?

As you again think of the values you identified in an earlier section of this chapter, what value would you honor most if you stepped up to address the issues of your own health?

What would motivate you to do it?

Will you commit to removing the trigger food from your diet that is impacting the quality of your life in order to support your own health and the health of your child? Who will you tell about this commitment?

CHAPTER 5 HIGHLIGHTS

THINGS THAT INFLUENCE YOUR ABILITY TO MAKE SUCCESSFUL CHANGE

- Change is difficult, no matter how much you believe it will make a positive difference in your life. As you change the diet of your family, there will be many outside and internal influences that will impact your success. Taking the time to notice where you are likely to stumble and identifying the personal and family strengths you can draw on will make a big difference in your success. This chapter reviewed a list of topics to consider along with some questions to support the identification of your own personal challenges and strengths. By taking the time to consider these topics before attempting to change your family's diet, you will significantly increase your chance of success.

1. Your definition of health for yourself and your family
2. The amount of stress in your life
3. Your past experiences with change in your life
4. The connection of your motivation to something you value
5. The balance and priorities of your busy life
6. The impact of your old stories and beliefs
7. Your ability to set healthy boundaries
8. Your ability to move past your own doubts and saboteuring voices
9. Your willingness to ask for help
10. Your willingness to address issues related to your own health

If you would like to purchase the workbook that contains all the questions from this book, go to my website at *www.foodsensitivechildren. com* for information. You will also be able to find additional resources and types of support listed there.

CHAPTER SIX

OKAY, HOW DO I DO IT?

Real-Life Story

John and Tanya adopted a little girl from Korea at the age of one. She was significantly underweight when they picked her up at the orphanage, and she had a constant runny nose. As soon as they returned to Canada, they sought the help of their doctor in identifying what they could do to make her well.

After many appointments with a number of specialists, John and Tanya were told that Sophie was intolerant to both dairy and gluten. They were stunned by the news and felt completely unprepared to undertake the significant challenge of adjusting her diet. Both of them worked full-time, and they had hired a Korean nanny to help them care for Sophie, so the job seemed overwhelming.

They decided to contact their local celiac society in order to learn more about what foods to feed Sophie and asked for a referral to a dietician. After a couple of weeks, they felt better prepared to cook for Sophie and even had found a few recipes that they liked, as well. What they weren't prepared for was all the other issues. John's parents were very critical of the diet and continued to try and feed Sophie inappropriate foods. Both Tanya and John had spoken to them about this, but they didn't seem to hear. Tanya and John prided themselves on being very self-sufficient, so they resisted asking for help from their friends. They began to feel more and more overwhelmed as they tried to balance their busy professional lives with the many needs that Sophie had. They both valued their health highly and wanted to offer the same gift to Sophie, but their lives seemed to be rushed, with little time for fun. Sophie's health improved on the gluten and dairy-free diet, but the older she got, the more she resisted sticking to it. As she went to preschool and saw the treats the other kids had, she had frequent tantrums and tried to grab their food. Tanya and John were stressed and concerned about Sophie and the future of their family.

In Tanya and John's story, the parents needed to ask for additional help to address the challenges they were facing. By considering how they could adjust their work schedules to make more time to be with Sophie and having stronger boundaries with John's parents, their lives would get easier. Both parents had limited time for exercise and the outdoor activities they used to do together, so designing a schedule that would allow time for fun is essential. Their lives underwent a very significant change when they adopted Sophie, and they had not fully acknowledged how different their lives were. They were united, however, in their love for Sophie and their commitment to creating a wonderful family, and this offers the motivation they needed to change.

Even when parents have identified the trigger food that is the likely cause of their child's symptoms, the journey can pose some challenges. If their lives are already packed full with other activities, finding time to shop in different stores or make more foods from scratch can seem overwhelming. Other family members often doubt the validity of their story and may be unwilling to make special concession for the children's diet at family functions. Parents may feel pressured to give in to the demands of others or their child and may find themselves repeatedly doubting their ability to make the changes successfully.

Successful diet change requires careful planning and organization. People must find a reason that is compelling and motivating to undertake the change and find support to make it work. By planning ahead and identifying the places where challenges might appear, the likelihood of success is dramatically increased. If you have not read through chapter five, I encourage you to go back and take the time to consider the questions before you actually begin to change the diet of your family.

This section of the book offers a step-by-step, proven plan to support your success as you change the diet of your family. Planning is essential, so read through the entire list and create the strategies you need before you begin.

THINGS TO DO BEFORE YOU BEGIN

Being organized and prepared before you begin to change the diet of your family is essential for success. Many clients hear me speak about the benefits of addressing food sensitivities on their children's health, and they leap into doing it immediately. While I love their enthusiasm to help their children feel better quickly, this rarely is successful and actually makes it more difficult to enlist to cooperation of children later on. If favorite foods are removed from children's diets before acceptable alternatives have been purchased, kids quickly refuse to cooperate with the changes.

Read all the steps below carefully, and take the time to plan how you will embrace these thoughts in your own life.

1. Purchase a journal or scrounge an unused notebook from your kids, and keep track of what you are doing and how it is going. In the beginning, small changes may be subtle, and you may miss them if you are not being very intentional about looking and writing them down. Be clear about what behavior

or symptom you hope will change once you remove the food, and then be intentional about looking for it every day. Be on the lookout, also, for other things that shift. Very often, behaviors and attitudes that parents assume were part of their child's personality turn out to be food-related. It isn't uncommon for a child to become more cooperative, stop cracking her knuckles, or be more organized, which may not have been the symptoms the parents were trying to influence by adjusting their diet.

2. Get very clear on the food that you will be removing from your family's diet by completing the questionnaire in chapter three. Remove only *one* food at a time whenever possible, as this is usually enough to take on in the beginning. It is important to make the least amount of change in your child's diet that is required in order to improve his or her health. It is impossible to predict how much improvement you will get from the removal of a food, so it is best to remove only one at a time and keep track of the results.

3. *Remove the food completely*—absolutely and totally. If you do not do this, you will sabotage your efforts and send your child on a roller coaster ride of symptoms. Each time you cheat, your child's symptoms will return, they will feel more miserable than they did before, and it will take several days for them to feel better. You must read every label until you are familiar with what brands to buy to ensure the food doesn't slip in by mistake.

4. Commit to removing the food for thirty days only. Don't imagine that it will be lifetime commitment, as this feels overwhelming. Begin with a short, manageable goal, and then re-evaluate what you will do after that.

5. Expect withdrawal. When the correct trigger food is removed from their diet, most children will experience symptoms of withdrawal. This usually means an increase in their previous symptoms for three to four days, which offers a clue that you are on the right track. This is important information, because many people mistake this for their child actually getting worse and abandon the process before they begin. It is important

to remember that once your child has gone through the withdrawal, their sensitivity to the food increases. Your child's body is beginning to heal, and it reminds him or her that it does want them to eat this particular food. This can be a difficult problem if you are not consistent with the diet, as the child will end up on a roller coaster of withdrawal, reaction, withdrawal, and reaction. Most people give up if this happens. Also, if your child cheats either on purpose or by mistake, this reaction helps you to notice what happens. It can be a wonderful motivator both for yourself and your child to help him or her adhere to the diet.

6. Take the time to sit quietly and plan your menus for the week, and if possible, for the entire month. Advance planning is the secret to success. Plan creative alternatives to the food being removed, and look for ways to match the texture and the flavour when you can. If your children love ice cream and you are removing dairy products, purchase a good soya, rice, or coconut ice cream as an alternative. By being sure that you have healthy substitutes in the house, both you and your children will be less inclined to reach for quick and inappropriate treats. Choose a time in your week to shop and purchase all the groceries required for the entire week.

7. *Create a plan that allows for a wide variety of food choices and that does not replace the food that has been removed with an over-consumed alternative.* I can't emphasize this enough. Many people simply replace loads of dairy-based foods with multiple daily servings of soya or apple juice, and eventually, the child becomes intolerant to these foods. In a perfect world, you would rotate the foods in your family's diet, with no single food being eaten more often than every four days. Don't be intimidated by the idea of this—simply do your best to ensure that a wide variety of foods make up your child's diet. This is also important, because we are not doing what many traditional physicians do, which is to follow a very restrictive elimination diet. We are removing only one trigger food, so it is essential to rotate the other foods in order to allow the digestive tract to heal. A variety of foods

also provides more of the nutrients your child needs for growth and good health. A workbook that contains a spreadsheet to help you create a rotation diet plan is available on my website at *www.foodsensitivechildren.com*

8. If you are removing a food from your child's diet that feels like the only thing he or she eats, don't despair. For a few days, they may push against you and refuse to eat many things, but they will eventually give in. When a food that is poorly tolerated is removed from the diet, the child's tastes will expand, and his or her body will again be able to help them make healthy choices. Most parents don't believe me when I tell them this, but trust me; it is true. Offer a wide range of interesting, healthy, and fun alternatives; place them on the counter in the kitchen between meals where your child can grab them as they go by and watch the snacks begin to disappear. You will be amazed at how your child will try foods they would never dare to taste before. It does require, however, that you stand your ground. Do not give in to your child's whining for an old favorite. Offer something else, and then take a shower to avoid the struggle!

9. Choose a time to begin that does not contain a lot of stress or new changes in the life of either your child or yourself. During the initial few days when the food is removed, your child will likely experience symptoms of withdrawal, so it is best to attempt these changes on a weekend or during a vacation when the pace of family life is slower and allows the child to have more calm and quiet. The symptoms that appear during withdrawal will mimic the symptoms being created by the food when it is eaten. It they are bothersome, you can help decrease them by giving your child a small, age-appropriate dose of Gravol.

10. Plan ahead for how you will respond when cheating or mistakes occur. No matter how vigilant you are, you will have a memory lapse now and then and will give your child a forbidden food by mistake. Your child will also make mistakes as they try hard to remember what is safe and what is not. When a trigger food is eaten after a period of time without it, an exaggerated response

will occur. If milk gave them a tummy ache, they will get a more uncomfortable tummy ache when they have been off it for week or so and then cheat. The symptoms that occur in these situations are one of the best ways to reinforce the reasons for being on the diet. Your child may share a treat with a friend at school or buy themselves some of the food that has been removed on the way home and experience symptoms either later that day or the following day. Remember that most food intolerance reactions are delayed, so if your child has a tummy ache, out-of-control behavior, or other symptoms, look back about twenty-four to thirty-six hours for the cause. When these situations happen, calm conversation is the best way to manage them. Point out to your child the connection between what they have eaten and the symptoms they are experiencing. Do not scold or criticize your child, but support and encourage their efforts. Stand firm, however, and don't give in. Stay connected to the bigger reason you are doing this.

11. Expect cooperation from your child and your family. While some situations may be awkward or difficult, do not let your kids turn the diet into a long sob story or a way to get excessive attention. A matter-of-fact attitude where you simply offer a fun alternative is a much better strategy. If they are visibly upset over a particular experience, allow them lots of space to express their feelings without criticism or judgment, but resist the temptation to give in. If you do, this will only reinforce that if they whine enough, they will be able to change your mind.

12. Teach your kids what they can and can't eat from the very beginning. Take them shopping with you, and have them read labels if they are old enough. Your goal is for them to make this a lifestyle, and they need to be educated about acceptable brands and choices when they are not at home.

13. Educate all the people in your life ahead of time. Tell your child's teacher if they are young, and enlist the cooperation of the friends whose houses they visit. Talk to grandparents, aunts, and uncles about what you are doing and why. If necessary, purchase a variety of non-perishable foods and leave them at

the places where your child visits regularly. For people who are willing to bake for your kids, give them some of your recipes—and even some of the ingredients, if you can. It is a special treat for a child to have someone other than their parents bake something special for them—something safe to eat.

14. Plan ahead how you are going to manage those people in your life who criticize what you are doing. There are bound to be people—perhaps even your doctor—who will be quick to remind you that your children's bones will likely crumble without dairy products or that they will be malnourished without bread. This is not true. If your child is going to be off dairy for an extended time, there are many good calcium and magnesium supplements on the market that kids love. When children eat a balanced diet with lots of fruits and vegetables, they will also get most of the nutrients their bodies need, including calcium. The improved health of your child will speak volumes about the benefit of addressing suspected food sensitivities—louder than anything you can say.

15. It is important to replace a habit that is being changed with another one rather than just leave an empty space. For example, if you normally have a Friday night pizza night, continue the ritual, but change the food that you eat. Enlist the kid's creativity in designing something else, and you will still have the opportunity for family connection that you developed—and the kids will quickly embrace the new idea.

16. Plan ahead for a celebration! Set a goal with your kids for a period of time that you will try the new diet, and then plan a special treat or event to celebrate how well you are doing. Keep in mind, however, that it takes a full four weeks of following the diet perfectly to determine how much benefit you will get. Depending on the age of your kids, create something fun they can look forward to. Younger children may need daily stickers, while teenagers might respond better to some cold, hard cash or the promise of extra use of the car. Be creative and ensure that the energy around the change is one of optimism and hope rather than struggle and frustration.

17. The very best strategy is to alter the diet of your entire house so that the foods being removed are not sitting in full view in the fridge. If you can't enlist the support of some family members or have not chosen to follow the diet yourself, be considerate of your child, and either eat offending foods when you are away from home or hide them in other places in the house. For young children, it is unfair to expect them to eat one food when a sibling or parent is eating the food they are desperate to have.

18. Be prepared for your own moments of frustration, disappointment, and doubt. There will be moments when you are tired and fed up with the idea and long to just give your child an old favorite but now inappropriate meal. Don't do it! This is the time to remember those values you identified earlier—the ones that remind you why you are doing this. If you need to, call a friend, take a break, go for a walk, order in, e-mail a friend—do whatever it takes to stick with the program. Even if you don't feel you have seen as much in the way of results as you had wished, seek help and support to redesign what you are doing rather than simply give up. If changes have not occurred, then it is likely that another food needs to be tried, so re-evaluate what your child is eating and develop a plan to remove that food instead.

19. If you decide to change your own diet, consider changing it before you ask your child to change theirs. A new diet is not always successful if both you and your child are experiencing withdrawal symptoms at the same time!

20. Arm your child with quick and fun answers to the questions of their peers about why they can't eat certain foods. Role-play with them before things happen so they will feel confident in standing up for what is right for them and not shy away and make up a story. This is wonderful practice for the years ahead, when you want your child to say no to drugs, alcohol, and peer pressure.

21. Be patient and gracious with yourself. Change takes time and small baby steps, so send your saboteur based voices of doubt on a permanent vacation and simply do your best. I do mean,

however, that you must do your best. Do not keep making excuses for why you won't do it today and allow yourself to consistently fall off the wagon, believing that you will do it "tomorrow". In my experience, tomorrow never comes, and you will never know what health might be possible for your child or for yourself if you do not follow the diet consistently for at least one month. My request is that you impress yourself with your effort, and that will be enough.

THINGS TO CONSIDER ALONG THE WAY

For some people, the journey seems easy, as the annoying symptoms resolve quickly and the child is miraculously better in a matter of weeks. For others, the ride is like a roller coaster, and it takes a little longer to find the blend of offending foods, life adjustments, balanced nutrition, and support. The age of the child also has a bearing, as children of different ages have varying degrees of willingness to cooperate. It is much easier to change the diet of an infant or toddler than a very independent teenager. Many teenagers and adults, however, are suffering with such significant symptoms that they are extremely motivated to change.

1. Find ways to motivate your child that are appropriate for his or her age. If you find your child losing interest or beginning to cheat, spend time with them to help them connect to why they are doing it. The values exercise that you did for yourself in chapter five is also helpful for your kids. For example, your teenager is likely to cooperate if you link diet changes to an improvement in his acne or elimination of his offensive digestive gas because of the importance of his social life to him. For a slightly younger child, information that his hockey or soccer skills might improve and make him an even more amazing player might do the trick. Toddlers just love to do things with Mom, so bake muffins and cookies with them, and they will eat them without any trouble at all. Creativity is the name of

the game, as well as persistence, so keep changing your strategy when the first ten don't work!

2. Expect occasional cheating! Sometimes natural consequences are the best teacher! Don't let yourself get angry—or, if you feel angry, resist the temptation to take it out on your kids. Encourage positive conversation around the topic, and try to enlist their support. Listen to their questions, and help them problem-solve solutions to the struggles they are having. But don't give in! If cheating continues and it is clear that they are not doing what you ask, a consequence may need to be created. If a child refuses to stop eating the lunches of others at school and continually ends up staying home with stomach aches, you may suggest they need to come home for lunch for a while. Create enough seriousness around the topic of the diet change that your child understands you are doing it to improve their health and happiness and not just to make their life miserable.

3. Persist with the diet for at least a month before you decide if it is working. The body takes a while to heal and cleanse the offending foods totally from the system. Trying it for a few days is not enough to decide if it is really going to work or not. This means a month where the diet is done almost completely perfectly and not a month with dozens of slip-ups and cheats. Each time you cheat, your child loses significant ground, so it is impossible to measure the success of the change.

4. Stay connected regularly with people who will support your efforts. Find those in your family who will acknowledge the courage of what you are doing and offer you their unconditional support. There is great power in having someone hold you accountable for the changes you are making, so the more people you tell about your story, the better. Keeping it to yourself as a guarded secret enables you to fall off the wagon without anyone knowing about it. The success rate when you have some other person to hold you accountable is about 97 percent, so it is worth sharing your journey. Check out my website at *www.foodsensitivechildren.com* for testimonials of people who have transformed their own health and the health of their children

if you begin to doubt whether it will work. You will also find additional opportunities for support listed there.

5. Don't give up if you don't seem to be getting results. Sometimes another food needs to be tried or a second food needs to be removed from the diet. If you don't get the success you were hoping for, take stock of your child's diet, and notice what food is being consumed on a daily basis or often enough to be the cause of symptoms. Refer back to chapter three and complete the questionnaire again to help you find the trigger food you may have missed. Remove that food for a month to see if you get the extra benefit you had been hoping for.

6. If your child's symptoms disappear and then resurface, you have likely added a food to their diet in a frequency that is creating symptoms. It could be a food they have always eaten, such as eggs, but now you have increased the quantity so they are eaten every day. It may also be that you added a new food to their diet that they are now eating often and that bothers them. It may be helpful to keep a food log for a few days so you can identify the food that has changed in your child's diet. The most common situation to occur here is with soya products. About 50 percent of the people who are intolerant to dairy are also bothered by soya. If you replace over-consumed dairy products with loads and loads of soya, it is very common for symptoms to return. It is important to rotate the milk alternatives that you use rather than focus just on soya.

7. Pay attention to the other parts of both your life and your child's. Food sensitivities are life related, and symptoms will often continue if the child is exhausted or stressed. Adjust the routines of your child's week so they aren't run ragged and ensure that they get to bed early enough to get enough rest. If some change is happening in your child's life and they seem stressed or upset, do everything you can to support them, but be sure they don't fall into the trap of looking for those old comfort foods. Be creative, and redesign those familiar comfort foods into something they can eat. When stress levels are high, our

motivation to slip off the diet is high—but so is the likelihood that eating the food will produce uncomfortable symptoms.

8. Cook foods and use recipes that your family is used to. Rather than try a whole bunch of new things, do your best to adapt your old standbys. There is much comfort for children in familiar routines, so make the least number of changes in the rest of their lives that you can.

9. Maximize your children's ability to choose. If you must restrict something that they want to have, offer them a number of acceptable alternatives so they get to choose on their own rather than have decisions forced on them. It will make your job much easier and decrease the frustrations they feel when you have to say no. This applies to children of all ages, including teenagers. The more you include them in your plans, the easier your life—and theirs—will be.

10. Continue to make conscious efforts to offer your child a wide variety of foods. Your child's health will improve more quickly if they eat many different foods so resist the temptation to allow them to eat only a few favorites. This also provides better nutrition and decreases the possibility your child will develop an issue with another food.

11. Be creative in the lunches that you make. Kids are very sensitive to the comments of their peers, so pay special attention to what is in their lunch bags. Enlist their ideas and be willing to create something that seems a little odd. Corn chips with salsa or spaghetti sauce are a favorite, and the other kids wish that their cool moms would give them that instead of sandwiches. When events like hot dog and pizza days appear, design something special with your kids. Perhaps you can bring McDonalds, Subway, etc. instead or make your own pizza or hot dog that they can eat. It is also possible for them to say simply that they "hate pizza" and eat a regular lunch, but if they make that choice, be sure to put in something special.

12. Find ways to manage birthday parties, sleepovers, and camp that work for your child. Depending on their age, they may be willing to have an alternative piece of cake from you, or they

may simply prefer to say no thank you. If hot dogs are being served that your kids can't eat, don't be afraid to encourage them to say they don't like hot dogs and simply have chips and pop instead. You can feed them the healthy stuff when they come home. The important thing here is to ask your child—don't assume you know what they want to do. Most parents are also very willing to cooperate if you give them a different milk to bake the cake with or ideas of acceptable snacks for your child that everyone will like.

13. If your child is going away to camp for an extended time, talk to the cook and find out what the menu contains. Express your willingness to send along substitutes that match what it is being served. I would also suggest that you talk to the camp director and ensure that your child will not be singled out in a way that will embarrass him or her. Find out ahead of time how mealtime will be organized and how your child will get any special food they need. Be sure to also send along loads of granola bars, fruit leathers, etc. in your child's bag so if the meals don't work out, he or she won't starve.

14. Don't forget to keep a diary. It is wonderful to be able to look back and be reminded of the symptoms and behaviors of your child before you changed their diet. It is easy to forget, and it can be a great motivator to be reminded just how difficult things used to be.

15. When you talk to your child or to other family members about the changes you are undertaking, a few techniques to help you successfully convey your message will be helpful. These skills are for use with preschool-age children and older, and you will find them useful with all the people in your life.

    a. Rather than assume you know what your child or other family member wants, ask nonjudgmental and curious questions. Simple statements that ask things like "What is important to you about not feeling different?" or "What is it about our son's diet you find most difficult" elicit more conversation than judgemental comments that sound like criticism and result in a breakdown in communication.

b. Create lots of opportunities to acknowledge the amazing qualities you see in your child as they adjust both to the diet changes and to the rest of their life. Be careful to acknowledge who your child is and not what he or she does. Acknowledgements that speak to the character of your child have the biggest impact.

c. Listen! Listen between the lines, and notice all the nonverbal signals your child is giving. If your child's behavior seems unusual or you detect something different in the tone of their voice, use a soft voice and a little physical touch to let your child know you are there. Create opportunities for them to talk, and then listen without judgement to what they are saying. Resist the temptation to offer solutions or comments that appear to minimize the situation. Acknowledge how your child feels and then ask what support you could offer.

16. Once your child is feeling better and you can see that the diet adjustments have made a difference, embrace your new eating pattern for life. It isn't a diet! It is a way of eating to promote the health and happiness of your child. Take time to read the chapter of this book about how feelings of grief and loss relate to changes in diet. While there will be moments when you'd love to abandon the entire thing, most days, you will celebrate the changes in your diet because of the difference they have made in your child.

17. If your experience removing one trigger food has resulted in very little change in your child's health or behavior, don't give up yet. First of all, make sure you are being honest with yourself about the job you did. Did you truly read every label and remove all of the food 100 percent? If you didn't, take a deep breath, and do it again—remove all the traces of the food in your child's diet. Be gentle with yourself, as this journey isn't easy, and simply connect to a value that really matters to you and give it another try. If you did it 100 percent, it might be that you have selected the wrong food, and the results reflect that. How do you know if the food you chose was not the right

one? If it was easy to give up, produced little or no withdrawal symptoms, had not been eaten almost every day, was not a food that bothered any other members of your family, and was not a food that your child craved, it likely was the wrong one. The solution is to repeat the process you did at the beginning by filling out the questionnaire in chapter three and examining the answers more closely. Do a little detective work, and then try again with another food.

18. If you are sure that the food you removed meets the criteria above and your child's symptoms are only slightly improved, it is possible that a second food is contributing to the symptoms. This is particularly common if dairy products have been removed and soya has been over-consumed. About 50 percent of the people who are bothered by cow's milk are also intolerant to soya, so both of these foods often need to be removed together. Examine your child's diet carefully, and look for another food that is being eaten every day in significant quantity. It is possible that because your child's health has been compromised for such a long time, his or her bowel is very inflamed, and another food is a problem. By carefully rotating the other foods your child eats after removing the trigger food, you can minimize the possibility of this happening. If there is a second food that appears to be an issue, remove it for a month, and see how much the symptoms improve. For information on adding foods back into your child's diet, refer to the next section.

19. If you fall off the wagon and find yourself overwhelmed and longing to give up, don't. Offer yourself lots of grace and patience for your efforts, and then reconnect to why you began the diet in the first place. What difference is it going to make in your child's future? What will be the long term-consequence of giving up now? Ask yourself what it is that is difficult at this moment, and problem-solve other ways of addressing it. Connect to something positive about the diet, and then gather yourself and begin again. If you need to, take your family out to dinner at a safe restaurant or find another distraction to change the energy of the situation.

ADDING FOODS BACK TO YOUR CHILD'S DIET

Once you have successfully removed the trigger food from your child's diet for a month, it is possible to try feeding it to them again to see what happens. However, if your child's symptoms were very challenging and they have experienced a dramatic improvement, I encourage you to be careful about adding the food back. For some of my clients, symptoms such as asthma or difficult behavior improve so much that the parents are simply unwilling to give their children the food again. The risk feels too difficult, and they are uncomfortable with the idea of potentially making their children feel very unwell for several days in order to prove that the food was the culprit. They are personally convinced of the connection between the trigger food and their child's symptoms and are comfortable with their decision to eliminate it for an extended period of time before challenging it again. Some physicians and family members may try and push you to reintroduce foods in order to be convinced, but do what you believe is right for your own child. If your child's symptoms have improved and their reaction to adding the food back is potentially life-threatening, do not do it on your own. Add the food back in an environment such as a doctor's office in order to have the medical support you need in the event of a problem.

If you decide to try giving your child the food again, pick the time that you do it carefully. Your child's symptoms are likely to return, so don't do it in the middle of your family vacation or before some special family event. Enlist the support of your child, and ask them what they would like to eat to test out the food. Many children are so excited to try adding the food back that they will tell you exactly what it is they want to eat. The idea of eating a piece of pizza or having a donut causes a sense of celebration for them, so embrace the energy of that so they truly savor the food as they eat it.

Remember that reactions due to food intolerances are often delayed and may not appear for twenty-four to forty-eight hours. Give your child a normal-size serving of the food on the first day, and then do not give them any more the next day. This will allow you to notice whether or not the small quantity that you gave produced any symptoms. If your child does not have any reaction, give them two servings of the food on the third day. Again, do not give them any additional servings the fourth day to allow time for a reaction to occur. You can repeat this pattern several times to see if there is a point where your child experiences a reaction. Food intolerances are also dose-related, and symptoms may only occur if the food is eaten in a large quantity or several days in a row. By following this process, you can decide whether or not the food needs to be eliminated completely from your child's diet or if they are able to tolerate small quantities now and again. Be honest with yourself as you undertake this process. I often see clients minimize reactions because they want to allow their child to return to eating the food, and children sometimes resist commenting on their symptoms so the food will be reintroduced into their diets. If you suspect your child is not being honest in telling you about symptoms they are experiencing, consider hiding the food you are adding back in a form where your child can not detect it.

When you choose a time to reintroduce the food into your child's diet, pay particular attention to the stress he or she is under and the pace of their life. Because food intolerances are closely connected to lifestyle, a reintroduced food may be poorly tolerated when offered during times of stress but may be tolerated better when the child is healthy and well-rested.

If the food that was eliminated was a major trigger food, it is highly unlikely that your child will ever be able to tolerate large or regularly consumed amounts of this food. This may be difficult to hear and produce a sense of loss so take time to read the section on grief in chapter four.

PARENTING IDEAS FOR MAKING SUSTAINABLE CHANGE

It can be overwhelming as a parent to try and figure out what books to read and what strategies to follow in raising children. There are thousands of parenting books on the market and many workshops you can attend to help you find strategies that address the unique needs of children at the various developmental stages of childhood. The best book that I have ever read is Gordon Neufeld and Gabor Mate's book, entitled *Hold On to Your Kids*.[31] The underlying theme of the book is that unless you create an environment where your children are lovingly attached and nourished by the adults who are caring for them, they drift off and become attached to their peers instead. It is a basic human desire and need to feel significant and attached to someone who loves you. If this need goes unfulfilled, children seek alternative places to feel they belong. The more they feel detached at home, the more they seek to attach to their inexperienced and immature peers. Their friends do not offer the nourishment and the safety they need, so the children become stuck in childhood and have great difficulty moving forward and becoming well-adjusted adults.

"Peer contact whets the appetite without nourishing. It titillates without satisfying. The end result of peer contact is usually an urgent desire for more."[32]

When I do workshops on the topic of food sensitivities, there are always many questions about how to parent children through these changes. When you meet resistance of some kind, you need some strategies to get past it. My husband and I have always tried to look at the big picture and focus on the values we were trying to develop within our family. Rather than get caught up in the challenges of the moment, we tried our best to step outside the emotion to regroup, and then create a plan from a calmer place. We certainly weren't always successful but things always went more smoothly when we were consistent. In the introduction of this book, our eldest daughter spoke of the impact that our commitment to our values had on her life. I had no input on what she wrote but was so very gratified to read about the values she felt were modeled for her.

Parenting is a challenging responsibility, and it is important that you find ways that work successfully for your own family. I encourage you to regroup often and take stock of how things are going. In my experience, it is easy to slip off track when life gets busy, and before you know it, your intentions of being consistent can disappear without you even being aware of it. As well, different children require different styles of parenting in order to reach the same outcome. Some push the limits and seem to forever be testing you to see how far they can go, while others have more quiet and cooperative dispositions, even as a toddlers. Parenting requires creativity, patience, and a good sense of humor.

A few of my personal thoughts on parenting:

Listen. Listen. Listen: True, compassionate, attentive listening is the secret to successful parenting. It fosters a close attachment between parent and child and is the foundation upon which we can support our children's growth into adulthood. Whether it is attuning to the needs of your crying infant, spending one-on one-time with each of your unique school-age children, or engaging your teenager in something he or she is passionate about, taking the time to truly hear what is going on in your child's heart and life helps your child know that you care.

When it comes to adjusting the diet of your child, the same principles apply. Listen to your child's thoughts and ideas, and engage them in meal planning and preparation. Use the topic to deepen the connection with your child and build a rapport with them as you problem-solve your way through the challenges that come up. When your child stumbles and finds a situation difficult, sit and listen until you can get a clear sense of what is causing the frustration; then problem-solve, together, how you might fix it. If your child understands you are doing what you believe is right for them because you care, they are far more likely to cooperate.

Be clear about what you value for your family and nurture it: One of the most successful exercises I do with my coaching clients is to help them create a list of the things that they value. Many of them have never really given concrete thought to the principles they use to make decisions and guide their lives. It is very powerful to create a list and to write it down in a place where you can refer to it when you need to make an important decision. This list helps offer clarity in the midst of decisions that are sometimes emotional and difficult.

The same concept is helpful in parenthood. If you are clear what you value for yourself, your family, and your child, it helps you make decisions in those moments when your child is pushing for something and you are feeling pressured to make a quick decision. It offers a framework around which you can design the future of your family.

Children also learn what values drive your decisions, and having clear values helps make your requests of them appear less random and unpredictable. They might not like your "no", but they understand why you said it. Children will also begin to embrace values of their own, which is a great activity to support. Point out the principles you see them using to make decisions so they can see for themselves if they are making choices for reasons that will design the lives they want. Doing things because everyone else is doing them rather than making choices that honor what they want looks less appealing when they can see what they are doing.

There is an entire section in chapter five that helps you identify the things in your life that you value. This is the information you will use to motivate yourself to stay on the diet when the going is difficult. Why are you attempting the diet, anyway? What difference are you hoping it will make to your child and to your family? What might be the outcome if you don't change the situation? All of us are motivated to change only when it matters. If someone else tries to convince you to do something and you don't believe it is worth it, you are less likely to be successful in your efforts. Usually, we change when we become so uncomfortable in our current situation that we are immensely motivated to do something about it.

Make home a safe place: I can't emphasize enough the importance of making your child feel loved, supported, and safe at home. This is important for all children, but is crucial for children who are having challenges at school and in life. If your child's behavior, learning difficulties, or health issues are making them feel different at school, your child needs a safe place to return to at the end of the day.

While all siblings fight and antagonize each other, it is best to have a zero-tolerance for children being mean to or critical of each other. It is your responsibility as a parent to model the standard of behavior in your home and to create an environment where your child escapes the challenges they may be experiencing in other places.

Changing your child's diet has the potential of transforming some of the challenges your child is facing in their day-to-day world. I have worked with many children where their bullying behavior, unusual nervous tics and twitches, severe learning disabilities, or even asthma that prevented them playing at recess have dramatically improved. It is difficult to make home a safe place if your child's behavior is out of control and they are constantly hurting their siblings. It is one of the most compelling reasons to give the diet a chance. Children's experiences in their world shape very dramatically how they feel about themselves. If they spend most of their days being yelled at, corrected, pushed aside, left out, or feeling alone, their self-esteem is harmed, and their confidence in who they are is shaken.

Model and expect respectful behavior: When people have asked me over the years what I think the answer is to a long-lasting marriage and raising successful kids, my answer is always the same—*respect*. If you raise your children in an environment where they respect themselves and respect others, it influences all the choices that they make. It isn't always easy to model it as a parent in your busy life, but it is important that you model it as often as you can. Even young children can understand the golden rule of "Do unto others as you would have them do unto you." Whether it is learning to ask for what they want in a polite manner as toddlers, treating their friends with respect in elementary school, or refraining from using pushy demands or rude behavior when asking for something from their parents as teenagers, kids learn from the boundaries and limits that are placed on their behavior.

The verse that says, "Children learn what they live" is also true, however. If we yell at our children, boss our spouses around, and complain about our neighbors and relatives all the time, our children will do the same. If you want your children to be respectful, you must treat them the same way—and apologize when you slip up.

This same environment of respect facilitates a peaceful change in the diet of your family. Talk together, be creative in your plans, don't criticize each other when someone slips up, and be patient with each other. Expect respect from your children for your efforts, as well. Do not allow them to sit down at the table and say, "Yuk, this is awful" after you have spent two hours trying to make a delicious dinner. This is not what you would want your son to say someday to his future wife.

Be consistent: One of the things children need most is a sense of security and safety in their relationship with you. If you are consistent and predictable in your expectations—no matter what the situation—your children will know where the boundaries of their lives are. If you are not consistent in what you expect from them, children are often reinforced to complain, whine, and moan over and over until you give in. This is exhausting as a parent and creates unnecessary friction between you and your children.

Once you make a commitment to change your family's diet, it is also important that you are consistent in your expectations of yourself and your family members. Model for them a sense of fun and adventure rather than stress or struggle to make honoring your commitment easier for everyone. Plan ahead well so you are not faced with situations in which you give in because you do not have the appropriate foods readily available. If your child cheats or makes a mistake, listen to their story and offer empathy, but do not support their choice. Help your child problem-solve how they could make a different choice next time. Again, you can offer your child room to express their frustrations without feeling pressure to give in.

Treat your child as an individual: One of the challenges of parenting a family with multiple children is adjusting the family routine to address the needs and wants of each individual. It is much easier to take all the kids to soccer practice together than it is to allow each child to choose and end up going to three different activities, but kids thrive when they do what they love. Part of listening deeply to your child is to honor their uniqueness. Rather than lump your kids together when you do things, help each child have a voice in the decisions, and ensure their choices are honored whenever you can.

Honoring your child's unique personality also means helping your child learn who they are. Take time to support what they love to do, and acknowledge their efforts, whatever the outcome. There is a significant difference between praising your child for what they do and supporting who they are and the effort they put in. We want our children to be internally motivated and to strive to be the best they can be for themselves rather than be driven by the outside accolades of others.

When you adjust the diet of your family, give lots of room for your kids' choices. Educate them in the grocery store, and enlist their help in cooking. Do your best to make the comfort foods that each child loves. If one child's diet is being restricted while the others' are not, be mindful of the situations that occur where the child with the restricted diet may feel excluded, and design creative ways to minimize that.

Do not, however, turn yourself into a short-order cook who caters to everyone's whims and picky choices. There is a balance here between feeding them well and allowing choice and feeling manipulated yourself. It is usually best to create a weeklong menu and give the kids some input. One child may not be so fussy about the chicken being served on Tuesday when he knows that his favorite, spaghetti, is coming on Wednesday.

Remember, everyone is learning: One of the most essential qualities of parenthood is a sense of humour. It is easy to get caught up in trying to make everything work perfectly, and this is usually a recipe for disaster. We are all learning how to be together, and it isn't always easy. Help your kids learn that mistakes are part of growing up, and the important thing is to learn from them so you won't make the same mistake again. As you work to keep a respectful and safe environment in your home, encourage your kids to laugh at themselves and find the light side of what happens. As our grandson happily announces when he or someone else makes a mistake or has an accident, "It's okay! We can fix it." Encourage them, too, to giggle at the places where you mess up. Be sure that your family is laughing together, however, and not at someone else or having fun at someone else's expense. Make lots of room for fun in your family, and don't let yourself get too serious about life.

Diet change in your family certainly contains many new things to learn. Take time to learn what you need to know before you begin rather than struggle in frustration along the way. Enlist the support of others who have done it before you, and try to find at least one other adult you can share your frustrations with. Share what you are learning with your kids, as well, as your ultimate goal is to raise kids who have a good knowledge of nutrition and can cook healthy food for themselves. Listen also for what the kids can teach you, as they often have wonderful ideas of things to try that you might never have thought of.

Create a village around your child: The idea that it takes a village to raise to a child is embraced by many cultures and families striving to keep their children attached to loving relationships. Parents can't be everywhere, so surrounding your children with warm, empathetic, and caring adults is a huge asset. This community offers your children safe places to go when they find life a little stressful and offers them the advantage of hearing different points of view. Building a village takes intentional effort and the creation of rituals and opportunities for people to get together. Whether it is your own adult friends and neighbours, the young adult children of people you know, or the circle provided by your extended family, children thrive when embraced by a loving community of caring adults. "We need to value our adult friends who exhibit interest in our children and to find ways to foster their relationship with them . . . . The greater the number of caring adults in a child's life, the more immune he or she will be to peer orientation." [41]

The power of creating a village of support around your family as you change your diet is huge. One of the biggest stumbling blocks for people attempting these changes is that they try to go it alone and refuse to ask for support from those who love them. Sometimes family and friends struggle to embrace the idea and offer criticisms instead, so don't include those people in your village. Seek out others who will help you stay motivated when the frustration builds and you'd like to quit the whole thing. People who love your children and want them to have bright futures will get behind your efforts and help in whatever way they can. Be clear in what you ask them to do, and be sure to express your appreciation for their efforts. A home-cooked meal that is appropriate for your family's sensitivities that you didn't have to cook yourself is a huge gift!

COMMON SUBSTITUTIONS FOR DAIRY, GLUTEN, SOYA, AND EGG

The process outlined in this book determines the individual trigger food for each individual child. It is not based on common problem foods, because I have seen too many times where the food that is the culprit is uncommon in the general population and would not normally have been implicated as a potential problem. The most common culprits are dairy, gluten, soya, and egg, but I have supported families to remove many other foods, such as chicken, raspberry jam, tomatoes, potatoes, sugar, artificial color, and corn. The best approach, therefore, is to follow the guidelines in chapter three and remove the food that is causing your child's unique symptoms rather than rely on a list of common offenders.

As you undertake the process of changing the diet of either yourself or your child, it is important to keep your overall nutrition in mind. No one ingredient, vitamin, mineral, or food group is more important than any other one. Balance in the key. Many children with food sensitivities are exceptionally picky eaters and limit their food choices to those containing the food that is the cause of their symptoms. This is actually an important clue in the identification of the offending food—the child craves it often and finds it difficult to give up. The same is true for adults, and it is often the parents' reluctance to give up a food they crave that prevents them from embracing the idea of doing it with their child. When the offending food is removed, it is common for children's tastes to expand and for them to be willing to eat many foods they previously refused.

People often ask me for recipes, and I seldom offer more than a very few because I want them to adapt recipes that are familiar to their children. The family will adjust more easily to the new diet restrictions if the ingredients in old family favorites are substituted rather than the choices being completely new. In the next section, however, I will offer some ideas for kid-friendly foods that are both delicious and fun. It is very important that you take time to create good alternatives for your children rather than simply offer them fruit and veggies every time. Homemade cookies and special treats are important comfort foods of home, so take the time to be creative and use the Internet to find interesting and different ideas. Simply search online for what you are looking for, and *voila*—a recipe will appear! Be sure to choose ones with five-star ratings so you know others have tried them with great success!

Below is a list of the words used to refer to gluten, dairy, soya, and egg in the common foods we all eat. It is essential that you learn these words and read the labels of the products that you buy. The idea might seem overwhelming at first, but very quickly, you will learn which products you can buy, and then you will not need to resort to the bother of label-reading. Because ingredients in foods do change, take time to reread the labels of the common foods that you buy every so often in case the manufacturer has made a switch.

Dairy Substitution

There is often some confusion about dairy products, as some people are intolerant to the protein and some people are only bothered by the sugar called lactose in milk. In children with consistent and significant symptoms, it is usually the protein in the food that is the issue and this requires removal of all foods that contain dairy. There are over thirty different proteins in milk, and any one of them can be the cause of the symptoms. If dairy products are the main trigger food for a child, is it very unlikely that they will be able to tolerate large amounts of dairy based foods for most of their life. Some people experience a true allergy to milk and can have very serious anaphylactic reactions in which their throats swell and they have trouble breathing. This is a medical emergency, and anyone with this allergy should carry an EpiPen and wear a medic alert bracelet. Most people, however, are intolerant to dairy products and experience very unpleasant but rarely life-threatening symptoms. If you refer to chapter two on allergies and sensitivities, you will find more information on this topic.

People likely to be bothered only by lactose are those who have had a serious bout of diarrhea or the flu. The enzyme lactase in the bowel is quickly destroyed when diarrhea occurs, and thus, the body is unable to digest lactose. This is why children and adults alike have only clear fluid juices when they have the flu because milk increases their symptoms. Their tolerance to dairy products usually returns, however, within a couple of weeks.

The other people who may be intolerant to only the lactose in milk are seniors. The amount of the enzyme lactase decreases with age, so their ability to tolerate dairy products is impacted. This is a very common problem in seniors, because they often have trouble cooking or chewing their food and resort to puddings, cheese, and cans of dairy-based Ensure. Many seniors suffer needlessly, and some even require physical care if their digestive symptoms become severe. Removal of dairy products from their diets often improves their symptoms very quickly.

List of words indicating that a food contains dairy products

This list was created from a wide variety of credible sources in order to produce a current and comprehensive list. Some good resources for this information are the website www.godairyfree.org and Dr. Janice Joneja's book *"Dealing with Food Allergies in Babies and Children."* Both of these are listed in the resources section of the book.

Ammonium caseinate
Acidophyllus milk
Butter
Butter fat, butter milk
Calcium caseinate
Casein
Casein hydrosylate
Cheese
Condensed milk
Cottage cheese
Cream

Lactose—common in some medications
Lactulose
Light cream
Malted milk
Margarines—some are dairy-free
Milk powder
Milk solids
Natural butter flavor
Potassium caseinate
Processed cheese
Quark

Cream cheese	Rennet casein
Cultured milk	Ricotta cheese
Curd	Sherbert
Custard	Skim milk powder
Delactosed whey	Sodium caseinate
Evaporated milk	Sweet dairy whey
Feta cheese	Whey
Half and half	Whey hydrolysate
Ice cream	Whey powder
Ice milk	Whey protein
Lactaid milk	Whipped cream
Lacoalbumin	Whole milk powder
Lactoglobulin	Yogurt

Dairy products are used as fillers in many products, so you must read the labels of everything. Crackers, cereals, breads, processed meats, cookies, cakes, pasta sauces, gravy, margarine, and almost any processed foods are suspect, so be careful. For things like bakery items, ask to read the label yourself. If taking a calcium supplement, read the label, as many are dairy-based.

Substituting for milk in recipes is very easy to do and rarely affects the taste or quality of the product that is made. Here are a few hints to consider:

1. The possible alternatives for milk at this point in time are soya milk, rice milk, almond milk, potato milk, and coconut milk. Additional products are always appearing, so be creative and try something new.

2. The best dairy-free margarine is Earth Balance. The company that makes Earth Balance also makes a spread that is soya-free, and it works very well in cooking and baking.

3. If you are using a milk alternative that is fat-free, the product you bake may be a little crumbly. Either add a little additional margarine or oil, or choose a milk alternative

with a higher fat content, such as regular soya milk or coconut milk.

4. Milk is an important ingredient to make products brown when they are cooking, so try not to substitute water as the only liquid. This is particularly important in things like pancakes, as they will taste fine but look rather pale. If you want to use carbonated water in order to help the product to rise and be lighter in texture, substitute only half of the liquid in the recipe with water, and use some other alternative, dairy-free beverage for the other.

5. If you are also replacing either the flour or removing an egg, it is very helpful to replace half of your liquid with a milk substitute and half of the liquid with a carbonated water. The carbonation produces a lighter product. I use this for all my baking.

6. If a recipe calls for buttermilk or sour milk, simply add about 1 teaspoon vinegar or lemon juice to 1 cup milk substitute to sour it, and then use as directed. If you need to replace yogurt, sour the milk as above, and then use slightly less liquid than the recipe calls for.

7. If your recipe calls for yogurt, you can purchase either plain or flavored soya yogurt instead. Some people tolerate goat's milk yogurt, but this is not a wise choice until you have eliminated all your symptoms and you are feeling totally well. Most recipes also work well with soft tofu in place of yogurt.

8. You can use milk substitutes for things like white sauces and gravies without a problem. If using soya milk, add a little bit of lemon juice to eliminate any soya flavor first.

9. Most recipes for puddings, etc. work best with higher-fat soya milks or coconut milk. Very low-fat soya, rice, or almond milk sometimes results in the product not thickening properly.

10. There are many different amazing ice cream alternatives on the market. There are multiple flavors that taste great and even such things as dairy-free ice cream sandwiches,

Creamsicles, and Fudgesicles, so you shouldn't have trouble satisfying your kid's sweet tooth. There is also one company that makes fruit juice-sweetened soya ice cream, which is wonderful and healthy at the same time!

There are very few cheese alternatives that are totally dairy-free, and the best one, hands down, is called Daiya cheese. It is produced in Vancouver, Canada and is dairy-, gluten-, and soya-free. It melts well on things like pizza and lasagna and tastes very good. Their website is *www.daiyafoods.com*

It is also possible to use fruit juice in place of milk, but be sure you don't use pineapple juice, as it impacts the baking process. The product you bake will have a different flavor and texture than with milk but often takes great. Some kids also prefer juice on their cereal instead of soya milk. Using orange juice in place of milk to make French toast was a favorite of our daughter's.

If you have a young, bottle fed infant less than a year who you believe has a dairy intolerance, it is important to seek the advice of a physician or other qualified health care professional. The diet of a child who is totally dependent on formula must be regulated carefully to ensure that it contains the appropriate nutrients. If you decide to switch to a soya based formula, check with your doctor. Also, if your child has colic and other symptoms with both milk based and soya based formulas, your doctor must prescribe a special formula to meet the nutritional needs of your growing baby.

If your breast feeding infant has colic and appears to have digestive complaints, symptoms often resolve if the mother removes dairy products from her diet. Dairy proteins are excreted in breast milk, so the mother must remove all dairy-containing foods from her diet. This can often produce a dramatic improvement in the baby's symptoms in a very short time. When the child begins solid food, they should not be given any dairy products until the age of two and even later, as it is very likely that this sensitivity will continue. It is also likely that the mother has sensitivity to dairy products and would benefit from removing them from her diet, even when she finishes nursing.

Gluten Substitution

There is often some confusion when people are trying to remove grains from their diet. Some people are intolerant to only wheat-containing foods, such as wheat and spelt, while others are bothered by all grains containing gluten. It is wise to remove all gluten-containing grains first and then, when symptoms have improved, gradually add back the other wheat containing grains.

Grains containing the protein gluten are the following: wheat, rye, barley, kamut and spelt. Some people find it necessary to remove oats, as well.

Some children and adults have very severe reactions to gluten that can result in serious weight loss and malnutrition. Infants may fail to grow and be chronically unwell. It is important that anyone with these symptoms be thoroughly investigated for celiac disease by a gastroenterologist. Do not attempt to manipulate your own diet without determining the medical cause first. If you are going to be tested for celiac disease, it is important that you remain on a gluten-containing diet until after the test is completed. A gluten-free diet will make the results inconclusive and inaccurate.

For many people, however, the test for celiac disease is negative, but they still continue to have symptoms. Although not diagnosed with celiac disease, many people are intolerant to gluten-containing grains and experience a tremendous improvement in symptoms when these grains are removed. There are a wide range of symptoms that can be related to gluten-containing grains, so be sure you complete the signs and symptoms check list in chapter one.

List of words indicating that a food contains gluten

This list was created from a wide variety of credible sources in order to produce a current and comprehensive list. Good resources for this information are the website www.celiac.com and Janice Joneja's book entitled *"Dealing with Food Allergies in Babies and Children."* Both of these are listed in the resources section of the book.

Barley
Bran
Bulgar
Couscous
Duram
Einkorn
Emmer
Farina
Fu
Gliadin
Graham flour
Gluten
Glutenin
Hemp (okay of not contaminated with gluten)
Hydrolysed plant protein (HPP)
Hydrolysed vegetables protein (HVP)
Kamut

Malt
Matzo
Medications—read labels or ask pharmacist
Modified starch
Oats, oat bran, oat fibre if contaminated
Rye
Seitan
Semolina
Spelt
Toothpaste—check with manufacturer
Triticale
Udon noodles
Wheat
Wheat berry, wheat germ
Wheat grass, wheat nut

Acceptable grains

Amaranth
Arrowroot
Bean and lentil flours
Buckwheat (in the rhubarb family)
Chickpea flour

Kasha (toasted buckwheat)
Manioc (cassava root)
Millet
Nut flour (any tolerated ground nuts)
Potato starch, potato flour

Coconut flour

Corn, corn starch, corn flour

Cornmeal

Dal

Dasheen flour

Flaxseed

Glutinous rice (sweet rice)

Gram flour (from chickpeas)

Hominy grits

Quinoa

Rice, rice flour

Sago flour

Sorghum

Soya flour

Tapioca

Tapioca starch flour

Teff

Gluten-containing flours are present in almost every processed food that you buy. You must read labels carefully for the ingredients you are trying to avoid. These flours are particularly common in baked goods of all types, crackers, cereals, cookies, processed meats, as thickeners in puddings and sauces, and as coatings on all types of meat and fish. The flours are also present in unusual places, such as French fries, so you must check with manufacturers or restaurant owners.

A few things to consider when substituting for gluten:

1. Cooking with gluten-free grains can be a challenge, and usually mixes of flours produce the best results. The recipes for the mixes below have been created through trial and error in many recipes in my family. Betty Hagman also has written a number of wonderful gluten-free cooking books and has developed some flour mixes that work well, too. Her books are listed in the reference section at the end of the book. There are also many recipes on the Internet to be found if you search for what it is you want to make.

MOM'S HEALTHY MIX
(I use this for most of my baking)

	9 CUPS OF FLOUR	12 CUPS OF FLOUR
Garfava bean flour	2 cups	2 2/3 cups
Sorghum flour	1 cup	1 1/3 cups
Cornstarch	2 3/4 cups	3 2/3 cups
Arrowroot starch flour	1/4 cup	1/3 cup
Tapioca starch flour	3 cups	3 cups

MOM'S FLOUR MIX
(I use this for things like sugar cookies)

	9 CUPS OF FLOUR	12 CUPS OF FLOUR
Rice flour	3 cups	4 cups
Tapioca starch flour	3 cups	4 cups
Cornstarch	2 3/4 cups	3 2/3 cups
Arrowroot starch flour	1/4 cup	1/3 cup
Potato flour	3 tablespoons	4 tablespoons

2. You must always add some xanthan or guar gum to the baking in order for the final product to stick together well. (Be aware that guar gum is corn based if you are removing corn from your diet). Add it to the dry ingredients and then mix well, as it is very sticky. You usually need about one half teaspoon per cup of gluten-free flour for a batch of muffins and cookies. Bread and pizza dough may require one teaspoon per cup of gluten-free flour. Depending on the other ingredients, you may need to add a little more. Recipes with sticky ingredients, like bananas, work well. If you are also removing eggs from the recipe, you will need to add more xanthan gum to compensate, even if you are using an egg replacer for the eggs.

3. There are many gluten—free products available in stores now, but unfortunately, they are often very expensive. I recommend

that you bake as many of your own things as you can and treat yourself to these specialty items only once in a while.

4. If you are looking for a list of products available in your area, check out your local celiac disease organization for resources. They are a wealth of information. There are also many websites on the Internet that offer well tested gluten-free recipes. If you search for things like "gluten-free muffins," you will also find websites galore that have many different recipes to try.

5. Bette Hagman has written a book on gluten-free bread-making that has loads of great recipes.[33] You can buy a bread maker or try your hand at baking your own in the oven. There are also a number of prepackaged bread mixes you can simply add liquids to and bake.

6. If you want to buy rice bread, the best bread currently available is made by Udi's and is found in the frozen food section of many stores. Their website is *www.udisglutenfree.com* There is also frozen, corn-based bread that is good and is made by Glutino, available at the same stores. Some bakeries make wonderful fresh bread, but if you are seriously allergic, you may need to be sure the bread is baked in a completely gluten-free bakery.

7. Both rice and corn-based gluten-free pasta are widely available in a range of shapes and sizes. The rice pasta holds its shape better and isn't as likely to turn to mush if you cook it too long. Many of the Asian pastas are rice based, as well, and usually less expensive.

8. For breading meat or fish, simply use gluten-free corn flake crumbs, ground corn chips, gluten-free rice cereal, or rice flour instead and add your own spices and herbs.

9. There are gluten-free pizza and pie crust mixes available, or you can make your own. I use corn flake crusts for most of my pies, as my kids prefer it, and make my own pizza dough from one of the flour mixes given here. You can also use frozen hash browns or mashed potato for pizza bottoms.

10. There are many snack foods and crackers that are gluten-free, but you must read the labels. Things like potato chips are

fine, but only if they are natural and do not contain any grain products.

11. Your local dieticians as well as nutrition resources on the Internet also offer great information about alternatives.

Soya Substitution

As prepared and premade food increases in society, so do the number of foods using soya as filler. Soya also is now often promoted as a healthy alternative to dairy, and there are many soya-based foods on the market. Almost 50 percent of the people bothered by dairy are also bothered by soya, so it isn't uncommon for people to have to remove both of these foods from their diets. As with dairy and gluten, it is essential that you read all the ingredients before you assume a food is safe.

List of words indicating a food contains soya

Edamame (soya beans)	Soya nuts
Hydrolyzed plant protein (HPP)	Soya protein
Hydrolyzed vegetable protein (HVP)	Soya protein concentrate
Miso	Soya sauce
Shoyo sauce	Tamari
Soya beans,	Tempeh
Soya flour, soya grits	Texturized vegetable protein (TVP)
Soya lecithin	Tofu
Soya milk	Vegetable broth—many contain soya

A few things to consider when substituting for soya:

1. Read labels carefully, as soya is used as filler in many places. Many vegetarian foods use soya protein as their base, so be particularly careful with these foods.

2. If you are vegetarian and avoiding soya and dairy, consult a dietician to ensure that your diet is nutritionally sound and healthy.

3. Asian cooking is often a good alternative for people avoiding dairy and gluten, but many Asian foods contain soya sauce, tofu, and miso. If you ask ahead of time, most restaurants can create alternative menu items by simply eliminating this ingredient. Don't avoid going. Just find a good local sushi restaurant where the people get to know you and are willing to be accommodating.

4. If you have an infant who you have placed on a soya formula that they do not seem to be tolerating well, see your doctor to replace it with a non-dairy, non-soya formula. There are some formulas available that are safe, but you must get a doctor's prescription to order them. Do not take your young infant off milk and soya and simply attempt to feed him or her solid foods and juice. Infants require more protein and fat, so seek the appropriate help.

5. If you have a colicky, nursing baby whose condition only improves slightly when you remove dairy products, you may also need to remove soya from you own diet. Many people bothered by dairy are bothered by soya, so try eliminating them both to see if it might help.

Egg Substitution

Eggs are an important ingredient in many baked goods, and removal of them can result in a crumbly product. There are several successful ways to replace the eggs in diets, and because of the popularity of vegan diets, there are many cookbooks and restaurants that offer delicious alternatives.

Eggs are one of the common ten food allergens and are not usually given to small infants until at least one year of age. The symptoms created by eggs can be numerous, and there are a small number of people who have severe, life-threatening reactions to them. If this is the case, be sure your child carries an EpiPen and wears a medic alert bracelet at all times.

Words indicating that a food may contain eggs

Albumen	Ovomucin
Egg Beaters	Ovomucoid
Egg white	Ovovitellin
Egg yolk	Pasteurized eggs
Emulsifier	Pavlova
Glaze on baked goods such as pies	Powdered egg
Many Asian rice dishes	Some custards and puddings
Mayonnaise	Vaccinations—some contain egg
Meringue	Vitelin
Omelets, quiche	Wines—some clarified with eggs
Ovalbumin	Whole egg

A few things to consider when substituting eggs:

1. Alternatives you can use to replace eggs in baking:
    a. One tablespoon flax meal, chia seed, or Salba plus 3 tablespoons hot water; let the mixture stand for 10 minutes, stirring occasionally, and use when thickened.
    b. EnerG brand egg replacer—purchase the powder and then simply add water
    c. 1 teaspoon double acting baking powder mixed with 1 ½ tablespoons oil and 1 ½ tablespoons water
    d. 4 tablespoons pureed tofu mixed with 1 teaspoon baking powder
    e. 1 packet gelatin and 2 tablespoons warm water
    f. 4 tablespoons of a sticky ingredient, like pureed fruit
2. Eggs are the binding ingredient in most baked goods. If you are removing eggs from your baking, recipes that contain sticky ingredients, like bananas and applesauce, often work best. Eggs may also be used to bind together things like meat loaf, hamburger patties, or the coating on chicken fingers so be sure to watch if you are ordering these foods in a restaurant.

3. Recipes that contain more than two eggs do not do well with substitutions. It is best to search for another recipe for the same food that requires fewer eggs.

4. If you are replacing an egg, I often find it helps to add ½ teaspoon guar gum or xanthan gum to the dry ingredients. It helps the end product to stay together better.

5. If you are removing the egg from the recipe, replace at least half of the liquid with carbonated water. This helps the product to be lighter and fluffier.

6. Eggs are often used to add shine and glaze to baked goods, like bagels and donuts, even if they have not been added to the dough itself. Be suspicious of shiny baked goods, even if someone tells you there are no eggs in the ingredients.

7. If you are making egg-free cookies, allow them to cool completely before removing them from the cookie sheet, as they may be very breakable. It is also helpful to line your cookie sheet with parchment paper.

8. Eggs are often used as a foaming agent in beers, lattes, and cappuccinos, so be sure to ask.

9. Many types of makeup, shampoo, and other personal products contain eggs, so be sure to read those labels, as well.

10. Many vaccinations contain eggs, so if your child's reaction is severe, be sure to tell your doctor before giving them any shots.

FAMILY FRIENDLY MENU IDEAS

Rather than offer specific recipes, I am going to offer meal suggestions, as this is the most common request that I get from parents beginning the task of changing their child's diet. I am a believer that the less you change, the better, so I would prefer to offer information on acceptable substitutions to make it easy to adapt your family favorites. Your children will be far more willing to accept the changes you are making if the pancakes you serve them and the birthday cake they have are as close to what they are used to as possible.

These ideas are based on the ones that worked well for my children. I needed to create meals for our family that avoided gluten, eggs, dairy, and spicy foods and yet tasted delicious. No small task some days but our kids have all grown up to be wonderful cooks and healthy adults which has made all that extra work worthwhile.

Breakfast

1. **Allowed cereal** with an allowed type of milk or juice. Add fruits such as blueberries and bananas as well as some nuts to increase the nutritional value and the amount of protein. Do your best to rotate the types of cereal and milk that you offer to avoid your family become overly attached to any particular one.

2. **Pancakes or waffles** using allowed flours and milk. If you need to avoid eggs as well, use one of the egg substitutes listed earlier in the chapter. Cook extra pancakes and use them in school lunches or as afterschool snacks. They are also convenient to warm up again the next morning when you are in a hurry. You can make your own fruit syrup by boiling frozen fruit and thickening it with cornstarch or other allowable flour.

3. **Crepes** made using pancake batter cooled very thin then filled with fruit and non dairy topping.

4. **Homemade granola** that you mix up with dried fruit, coconut, nuts, and allowable grains and bake in the oven. Add some honey and oil and simply bake it at 325 degree Fahrenheit until it is crispy. Serve with soya yogurt, applesauce, or milk.

5. **Potato latkes**—most recipes use only grated potatoes and onion and are quick and easy to make. Most common cookbooks have a recipe and the Internet is a good resource, as well.

6. **Breakfast wrap** using a wheat, rice, or corn tortilla. You can fill it with anything at all—scrambled eggs and bacon, fruit and peanut butter, dinner leftovers, sliced meat, or allowable cheese. These can also be wrapped in foil and sent to school as lunches. Our kids loved tortillas spread with peanut butter, rolled around a banana, and then cut into bite-size pieces.

7. **English muffins with eggs, ham**, etc. on top. There are a number of companies that make good gluten-free English muffins and bagels that work well.

8. **French toast** that can even be made the night before and then toasted. Kids love them cut into fingers so they can dip them in syrup or honey. You can use juice, such as orange juice as the liquid, to give it a different flavor. If you need it to be egg-free, simply add one of the egg substitutes to the juice or milk along with a little vanilla and fry it in a frying pan.

9. **Leftovers** from dinner the night before. Depending on what you are having, cooking extra dinner can make a perfect quick breakfast. Kids usually love things like pizza or spaghetti with meat sauce in the morning.

10. **Cinnamon buns** made from frozen bread dough that is dairy and egg-free cut in strips, sprinkled with cinnamon and brown sugar, and rolled up. Allow them to rise for an hour and then bake. This is usually best done the night before, but delicious as a treat when you need a dairy-free and even an egg-free treat.

11. **Hot cereal baked overnight** in the slow cooker. You can add fruit, nuts, seeds, and a mixture of grains along with some honey and vanilla, and it will be hot and ready to eat in the morning.

12. **Breakfast pizzas** with ham, pineapple, tomato sauce, and allowable cheese made on English muffins or tortillas.

13. **Cut-up fruit that can be dipped in a nut butter mixture**. Combine ½ cup nut butter, 2 tablespoons of applesauce or other fruit sauce, and some soya or coconut milk together until you get the desired consistency. You may also add a little cinnamon. If you prefer, you can simply have them dip fruit in regular nut butter. Kids love this as a snack, as well.

14. **Homemade muffins**. Nothing beats the sweet taste of homemade muffins when you are in a hurry in the morning. Bake them in large batches and freeze them in small batches for quick microwaving. There are many recipes on-line that will help you make delicious muffins that use the grains, milk, etc. that your family needs.

15. **Omelets, scrambled eggs, fried eggs**, etc. These are quick and easy for kids in the morning as long as your child tolerates them.

16. **Rice pudding** made the night before using coconut milk, raisins or other fruit, and honey. The coconut milk makes a delicious flavor, but you can use any type of milk or juice.

17. **Fried peanut butter and banana sandwiches**. These are delicious and different. You can also send them for lunch.

18. **Cornbread or Johnny cake.** This is easy to make with alternate flours and can be served warm in the morning with syrup or jam. There are also a number of good gluten-free corn bread mixes.

19. **Regular toast** and nut butter with jam or honey. Try your hand at making your own gluten-free bread using Betty Hagman's bread cookbook or buying one of the ready-to-mix packages of bread.

20. **Hash browns mixed with bacon, egg**, or just on their own. You can also use hash browns as the base for other toppings, such as cheese or ham, and bake them in the oven.

21. **Stewed fruit**, such as apples, pears, peaches, etc., cooked on the stove or baked as a crisp in the oven. For a topping, mix 1 cup brown sugar, ½ cup allowable margarine, and 2 cups uncooked oatmeal, quinoa, or other flour mixture and bake.

22. **Fruit smoothies** made with fresh or frozen fruit and either juice or an allowed type of milk. You can also add a handful of nuts or a tablespoon of nut butter to increase the amount of fat and protein.

Lunch

1. **Homemade pizza pockets** made from frozen bread dough cut in strips; spread with tomato sauce, meat, or allowed cheese; and then rolled up and sealed at the edges. Allow to rise and bake in the oven until the bread is done.

2. **Corn and rice chips with salsa and hummus** as dips.

3. **Enchiladas**—layer the tortilla with salsa, allowable cheese, avocado, beans, etc. and then bake in the oven.

4. **Homemade soup** with allowable ingredients.

5. **Slices of meat rolled around pieces of cucumber**, carrot, pepper, or fruit. You can also spread a little mayonnaise or mustard on the meat before you roll it. You can also use other appetizer ideas, such as smoked salmon rolled around cooked asparagus. Kids like bite-size pieces of food.

6. Corn, rice, or wheat tortilla filled with fruit or vegetable salsas and meat. These are great to wrap and take to school.

7. **Rice wraps or lettuce wraps filled with meat or veggies**. For rice wraps, follow directions on the package to soften them before filling with veggies and meat. For lettuce wraps, cook some meat; chop up veggies, such as carrots and zucchini; cook some rice or sprouts; and then fill the long, endive type of lettuce leaves. Use allowable salad dressings or teriyaki sauce on top. You can use tiny lettuce leaves to make these into appetizers.

8. **Pizzas** made with a number of different types of crust. You can use corn, wheat, or rice tortillas; grated hash browns pressed into a pizza pan; or homemade pizza dough. There are lots of gluten-free pizza dough recipes on the Internet. Spread the crust with an allowable topping, such as tomato sauce, spaghetti sauce, or even hummus or salad dressing if your child can't eat tomatoes. Top with veggies, meat, pineapple, etc. and whatever cheese your child is allowed. Kids love to help make their own pizzas.

9. **Muffins** made with protein ingredients, such as nut butters or cheese, or buns filled with chopped ham or turkey. Combining these with some veggies and dip makes a complete lunch for a child.

10. **Gluten-free wieners and sausages**. Many delis now make their own sausages and wieners that contain only pure meat without any fillers. Regular hot dogs most often contain milk, but often the pure beef ones are okay. These can also be added to homemade baked beans for more nutrition.

11. **Burgers and fries** are a common favorite. Make your own patties, if you can, from ground turkey or beef, and add any allowable ingredients your child likes, such as a little ketchup, onion, Worchester sauce, or allowable cheese. You can also slice your own potatoes or sweet potatoes to make the fries. Simply cut them into a pan, toss with a little oil and bake.

12. **Leftovers from dinner** the night before. Just make extra spaghetti, casserole, etc. and save yourself time the next day.

13. **Rice, corn, or wheat pasta** with either safe, store-bought sauce or homemade sauce. You can add some grated veggies to the sauce along with some meat to increase your child's vegetable consumption. You can also make some homemade pesto and toss that with your noodles.

14. **Tacos** with refried beans, lettuce, guacamole, salsa, and allowed cheese or sour cream. My kids' favorite was when I made a mixture of ground beef, spices, onions, and salsa with soya cheese on the top and then baked it all in the oven until the cheese melted. They then used it as a dip with corn chips. I usually allowed each child to make their own in an oven proof bowl so they could select their own toppings.

15. **Tuna puffs** made from refrigerated Pillsbury Crescent rolls cut in half and pressed into small muffin tins. I filled them with tuna, celery, onion, allowed cheese, and either mayonnaise or allowed salad dressing, then baked them in the oven. This is dairy-free but not gluten-free.

16. **Salad** made from any combination of vegetables, fruits, and grains. Kids often prefer their veggies plain with a dip so give them the choice. The possibilities for dips are endless. You can use simple hummus, use a prepared salad dressing, combine mayonnaise or yogurt with herbs or check your cookbooks for other ideas. Dips are a great way to increase your child's intake of protein as well as get them to eat their vegetables.

Dinner

1. **Many of the suggestions in the breakfast and lunch** sections also work well for dinners.

2. **Vegetarian stews made with beans and lentils**. If your child prefers a more pureed consistency, simply use your hand blender to break down the larger pieces.

3. **Chicken fingers** can be made by dipping small pieces of chicken in ground corn flake crumbs, gluten-free cracker or bread crumbs, or allowed cereal crumbs. Add some spices and herbs and mix well before dipping. You can dip the chicken in melted butter, oil, or water to help the crumbs stick better. Just bake at 350 degrees for about 20 minutes until they are crispy.

4. **Roasted or barbequed meat** served with steamed veggies and either rice or potatoes makes an easy meal that kids usually love. I often allowed the kids to dip their meat in a healthy, low-fat, low-sugar salad dressing, as they loved the idea of dipping by themselves.

5. **Stir fries** of all kinds is a great way to clean out the fridge. Use up whatever veggies and even fruits you have, and add some leftover meat and nuts. To increase the flavor and to avoid soya sauce, use a healthy salad dressing, or thicken a juice such as orange juice with a little corn starch to make the sauce.

6. **Pasta** with a variety of sauce ideas. You can use the traditional spaghetti sauce or simply toss the noodles with some herbs and butter and serve as a side dish. You can also use grated or peeled zucchini or spaghetti squash as the "noodles" to increase the veggies your child eats. You can also buy a wonderful gadget called a Spirooli at many Asian and kitchen stores that turns vegetables into long strands that look like pasta and other fun shapes.

7. **Main course salads** can be a hit with kids if the kids get to choose what they put on their salads. Simply cut up a wide number of vegetables and tell your kids they need to pick at least three colors. Add some cut-up chicken, beef, nuts, or chickpeas to round out the nutrition.

8. **Takeout or homemade sushi**. Sushi is often a great choice, as it rarely contains dairy or gluten. If you are avoiding soya, simply ask to have it made without soya sauce.

9. **Stuffed baked potatoes**. Simply bake the potatoes first and then offer a variety of things to fill them. Finely chopped vegetables, grated cheese, salsa, refried beans, etc. all work well.

10. **Stone Grills** are a favorite in our house and can be bought at many kitchen stores. Rather than having a fondue, you simply heat up these grills in the oven and then place them in a rack over a flame. You then grill meat and veggies at the table. This is usually great fun for everyone and feels like a special meal, even though what you are cooking is simply plain meat and veggies. You can either make or buy a number of healthy dips, as well.

11. **Casseroles** are an easy way for busy parents to plan ahead. Simply layer veggies, rice, or potatoes and meat in a casserole dish and bake. Our kids loved layers of wild rice, broccoli, chicken gravy, and chicken topped with soya cheese. I baked it the night before, and it was easily warmed up the next day. Be creative and use up your leftovers, as well.

12. **Homemade chili** with corn chips or homemade corn bread is also an easy make-ahead dinner. There are also store-bought organic chilies available for a quick meal.

13. **Baked chicken** is easy if covered with a simple sauce, such as a mixture of honey, barbeque sauce, and garlic; a sauce made of equal parts of orange juice and chicken soup; or simply a rub of oil, lemon juice, and herbs.

14. **Foil dinners** are a favorite camping meal and be easily adapted to be enjoyed at home. Take two pieces of heavy-duty aluminum foil and rub with oil. Place sliced chicken, sliced potatoes, onions, and other veggies on the foil with a little oil and some herbs and wrap tightly. Bake in the oven or on the barbeque for about 25 minutes. These are easy to prepare the night before and simply place in the oven when you get home. Be sure to cut the meat and the potatoes small so they cook evenly.

15. **Hamburger pie** is easy to make and usually is a huge hit with kids. Simply take about a pound and a half of ground meat and mix it with a little onion, allowable bread crumbs, and ¼ cup of a liquid such as tomato sauce, spaghetti sauce, or gravy. Press into a pie plate. Fill the centre portion with cooked rice mixed with whatever finely chopped veggies you want and more of the liquid you used for the crust. Press down well and cover with grated allowable cheese if you wish. Bake for forty minutes at 350 degrees.

16. **Impossible pie** is another quick meal you can cook the day before. Brown about a pound of meat with some onions, garlic, and whatever grated veggies you would like. Spread mixture into the bottom of a pie plate, and level it carefully. Mix ½ cup of any milk substitute, three eggs, and one cup of any type of flour until mixture is smooth and pour this over the meat mixture. You can add some grated allowable cheese if you like. Bake at 350 degrees for about 30 minutes.

17. **Individual meat loaves** are a simple menu for young children. Bake your favorite meat loaf recipe in muffin tins. Mix up a little ketchup with some brown sugar and spoon over loaf tops before baking. The cooking time is reduced to about 20 minutes because of the size, and you can hide loads of veggies in the meatloaf; your kids won't even notice.

18. **Pastas of all shapes** and sizes are easy to find in most grocery stores now, so it is possible to recreate most pasta dishes, such as lasagna. Simply layer the noodles with sauce, meat, allowable cheese, and soya sour cream (if tolerated) and bake.

19. **Haystacks** was another family favorite. I cut up a wide range of veggies, such as celery, green onion, peppers, and zucchini, and placed them in small bowls. I then put out bowls of fruit, such as pineapple and mandarin oranges, as well as some coconut, ground nuts, and chicken. I cooked some rice, and the kids simply put rice on their plates and covered it with whatever other ingredients they wanted. They then poured hot gravy over the top made either from thickened chicken broth or a store-bought, healthy alternative.

20. **Hearty soups and stews** of all kinds make great make-ahead dinners. If you serve fresh allowable breads or muffins with soup, kids often like to dip them in the soup.

Snacks and desserts

1. **Many of the items listed previously for breakfast, lunch, or dinner** also make great snacks.
2. **Nuts and bolts** which is simply a mixture of different types of cereals and nuts combined with some oil and spices and baked in the oven. Check the Internet for a recipe that will suit the tastes of your family members. Kellogg's Crispix cereal has a recipe on the box.
3. **Rice Krispie squares** are always a favorite. Add some chocolate chips, nuts, peanut butter, etc. to increase the nutrition. You can also spread the Rice Krispie mixture out very thinly on a cookie sheet and cut it with cookie cutters into shapes for a holiday season, such as Christmas. You can also mould them into shapes and decorate them with icing, candies, etc.
4. **Leftover waffles or pancakes** make a great snack when spread with a nut butter and jam.
5. **Veggies and hummus** are great school snacks for young kids. Cut the veggies into safe sizes and interesting shapes.
6. **Fruit with the nut butter dip** mentioned in the section on lunch.
7. **Homemade or store-bought granola bars**. There are many easy recipes to make them yourself so you can add a large number of healthy nuts and seeds.
8. **Homemade or store-bought ice cream alternatives**. There is now a wide variety of non-dairy ice cream made from rice, soya, almond, coconut, and cashews. Many are not sweetened with sugar and offer a special treat for a child if dairy has been removed from his or her diet. There are also a number of dairy-free ice cream bars. You can make your own ice cream sandwiches by putting an allowable ice cream between two gluten-free or regular cookies and freezing.

9. **Ice cream pizzas**. Simply mix some allowable crumbs with melted butter and press in a pizza-shaped pan. Partially melt some dairy-free ice cream and spread it over the crust. Allow your child to help you decorate the top with suitable candies, sprinkles, etc. and then place back in the freezer. This works well as a birthday cake either for your own child or as something to take to someone else's party. You can also press the ice cream into a normal-sized cake pan and decorate it so it matches the ice cream cake being served at a party.

10. **Ants on a log** are an old standby. Simply put nut butter on a piece of celery and place raisins along to top to look like ants.

11. **Smoothies** are a great way to add some additional fruits and vegetables into your child's diet. The possibilities are endless. You can also add a little nut butter to the mixture for some additional protein. Simply put some fruits and veggies in your blender and then add some type of liquid (milk substitute, juice, coconut milk) and blend. You can use frozen fruit or simply add some ice cubes to make it cold.

12. **Cupcakes** made with alternative flours often bake well in small muffin tins rather than large ones. Kids love to be able to have four cupcakes, even though they are little. The same goes for baking muffins, so bake them bite-size, as well, and kids are more likely to eat them.

13. **Puddings** are an easy dessert to adapt to most types of diets. Rice pudding can be made with coconut milk or other alternatives with some dried fruit, such as raisins, added for more nutrition. Use brown rice to increase the nutrition. Many of the commercial puddings are made with corn starch, and you can make your own easily from scratch using a different thickener, as well. Most puddings do best when you use a high-fat milk substitute, as they often don't thicken very well if you use a low-fat variety. Coconut milk works extremely well and tastes delicious!

14. **Pies** of all kinds are easy to adapt to a special diet. For the crust, you can purchase a gluten-free pie crust mix, make your own from allowable flours, or use crumbs such as cornflakes or

other cereals and nuts. If using crumbs, use 1 ½ cups crumbs, 2 tablespoons sugar, and just over 1/3 cup melted butter or margarine for each pie. For the filling, simply use whatever fruits you want or substitute for the milk, etc. if you are making something like a pumpkin pie. If you need to add a thickener to your fruit pie, you can use corn starch, tapioca starch, or potato starch, as well as whatever gluten-free flour mix you have. For a topping, it is easiest to make a crumble type of crust with ½ cup margarine, 1 cup brown sugar, and 2 cups gluten-free flour or oatmeal. You can also add some ground nuts. If you prefer to make a crisp, place the fruit in a glass pan with some sugar (if required) and some thickener, and cover with crumble mix before baking.

15. **Homemade chocolate bark** is easily made by melting dark, dairy-free chocolate and then adding some type of nuts. Spread the mixture on wax paper to cool, and then break into pieces. You can also add ground-up candy canes at Christmas. Many kitchen stores sell some wonderful chocolate molds, and you can make chocolates with your kids. Melt the chocolate, pour into the molds, and remove when the candies cool. This is a favorite holiday event for kids and enables them to have special chocolates that meet their diet requirements—as long as you buy the correct chocolate.

16. **Cake recipes** using regular wheat flour can easily be adapted to be gluten and dairy-free. The Internet is loaded with recipes that are both delicious and easy. Gluten-free cakes that use ingredients such as banana and applesauce work very well because of the sticky texture of these foods.

17. **Finger Jello** made from juice and cut with cookie cutters is a fun afternoon activity for kids. Mix 1 ½ cups juice, ½ cup water, and 2 packages unflavored gelatin, and allow mixture to sit for a few minutes until the gelatin softens. Heat slowly on the stove until the gelatin is completely dissolved. Remove from the heat and add another 1 ½ cups juice. Pour into a shallow pan, and allow it to cool in the refrigerator. Cut with cookie cutters. You can also make finger Jello with commercial Jello

by mixing 1 (6 oz.) package of Jello with 2 ½ cups water and 2 packages unflavored gelatin.

18. **Homemade trail mix** can be made with your kid's help and stored in small bags in the fridge as long as your child is old enough that he or she won't choke.

19. **Store bought gluten free mixes** are available to make cookies, cakes, brownies, bread and other treats. You can also purchase a wide variety of products over the internet.

CHAPTER 6 HIGHLIGHTS

THINGS TO DO BEFORE YOU BEGIN

- It is important to carefully plan how you are going to adjust your family's diet before you begin. This section contains a long list of ideas and ways to help you get organized before you start.

THINGS TO CONSIDER ALONG THE WAY

- Once you begin to remove the trigger food from the diet of your family, you will inevitably hit a few challenges and hurdles. This section offers problem-solving ideas and suggestions on how to successfully navigate the diet change in order to obtain sustainable change.

ADDING FOODS BACK TO YOUR CHILD'S DIET

- It is never our goal to have children off more foods than absolutely necessary to maintain their health.
- Adding foods back must be done thoughtfully and carefully in order to get accurate information about what the trigger food might be.
- Foods must be added back one at a time and your child's reaction must be monitored for several days in order to determine if the food is tolerated. The amount of food given is also gradually increased, as food intolerances can be related to the quantity of food eaten.
- Foods intolerances are also related to the child's mood and stress level, so foods should not be challenged if the child is ill or under excessive stress.
- Food allergies that produce life-threatening reactions must be challenged under the watchful eye of a physician in an office prepared to offer medical assistance if it is required.

PARENTING IDEAS TO MAKE SUSTAINABLE CHANGE

1. Listen, listen, listen.
2. Be clear about what you value for your family, and nurture it.
3. Make home a safe place.
4. Model and expect respectful behavior.
5. Be consistent.
6. Treat your child as an individual.
7. Remember, everyone is learning.
8. Create a village around your child.

FOOD SUBSTITUTIONS FOR DAIRY, GLUTEN, EGG, AND SOYA

- There are many foods that potentially create symptoms for individual people. While dairy, gluten, eggs, and soya are very common, it is possible for people to be bothered by any foods in their diets. This section explains how to successfully replace dairy, gluten, soya, and egg in foods.

FAMILY FRIENDLY MENU IDEAS

- This section contains menu ideas for breakfast, lunch, dinner and snacks that are kid friendly.

CHAPTER SEVEN

CHILDREN WITH AUTISM AND OTHER DISABILITIES

FOOD SENSITIVITIES AND THE AUTISM SPECTRUM

Real-Life Story

Charlie and Carolyn are at their wit's end. Their son, Jason, who was diagnosed with autism at the age of two, is now facing a multitude of challenges at the age of nine that they feel unprepared for. He does not speak at all and can become very persistent and aggressive when they fail to anticipate his needs. He attends a regular elementary school in his small town, but finding appropriate support workers has been a difficult task. Often, for weeks at a time, Jason must remain home with his mom, because he is unable to attend school without a trained companion. This requires Carolyn to take time off from work, which stresses the family budget and makes it even more difficult to pay for the wide range of therapies that Jason needs. The family travels often to Vancouver to see various specialists and therapists in order to design a comprehensive program that they hope will improve the level of their son's functioning. They worry continuously about his future and are frustrated by the fact that, despite the many therapies they have tried, Jason has no verbal skills

Jason's story began in infancy, when he cried almost continuously and often refused to nurse. Finally, in desperation, his mother switched him to a cow's milk based infant formula in the hope it would improve his gassy tummy and allow her a few hours' break in the day, which she desperately needed. The change in milk seemed to make matters worse, and Jason cried continuously and slept for only a few minutes at a time.

As Jason grew through toddlerhood, he always seemed more withdrawn than his peers. He had no interest in socializing and preferred to play with the wide variety of household objects that he could spin around over and over. He was plagued by chronic ear infections requiring antibiotics as a child and seemed to get diarrhea from almost all the foods he ate. His diet became more and more limited, and Carolyn found herself trying to bribe him to eat by offering him plain noodles or cheese strings at every meal.

By the age of four, he was withdrawing more into himself and refused to eat almost all the foods his parents offered him. His diet consisted of plain, cooked pasta with no sauce and pizza from which most of the topping had been scraped off. Multiple trips to professionals specializing in autism had helped the family develop some strategies to improve their son's eye contact, but they had seen little improvement in his verbal, language, or attention skills.

Charlie and Carolyn did their best to stay on top of the current literature, as they were both determined to find some way to help Jason communicate verbally. One weekend, as they attended a National Conference on Autism in Vancouver, their answer appeared. A chance meeting with me as I sat in the chair beside them at the meeting sparked their interest about the impact food might be having on their son. After over an hour of conversation, they were committed to giving it a try. They came to understand that gluten could be a significant reason for their son's brain fog and inability to formulate words. Armed with packages of rice pasta and a recipe for gluten-free pizza dough they returned home.

Three weeks later, the results were nothing short of miraculous. Jason had willingly eaten the alternative foods and had begun to speak in full sentences. His diet had expanded and he often asked for a number of fruits and vegetables. Because he could communicate his needs more appropriately, his aggressive behavior diminished and the entire family was able to create a more positive and peaceful energy in the home. Jason's experience at school became more positive, as he was less aggressive with his peers, and he seemed to be more receptive to the behavior therapy that was being used to help him. Jason's progress in all areas of his life continued to astound all those who had worked with him, and they were hopeful that this progress would continue as long as he stayed on the diet.

CAUSES OF AUTISM

The spectrum of abilities and challenges in children with a diagnosis of autism is wide and varied. The learning, behavioral, and social development of these children can be anywhere on the spectrum from minimally delayed to significantly impaired. It is also believed there are hundreds of children with autistic-type behaviors who are not identified at all and grow into adulthood facing significant learning, social, and behavior challenges.

Research suggests a very strong genetic link in autism, and it is not uncommon to see more than one child—usually boys—in a family with the disorder.[34.] Research continues in an effort to search for a specific gene that may help to identify autism before a child is born. There is, however, much controversy about the factors that trigger children to develop the actual symptoms of autism, and there is still a great deal of research to be done in this area. Current areas of research focus primarily on the link between vaccinations and autism, exposure to environmental chemicals, such as mercury, both during pregnancy and after delivery viral infections, food sensitivities and an imbalance of vitamins and minerals in the body.

`In her book *Gut and Psychology Syndrome*, Dr. Natasha Campbell-McBride addresses what is believed by many professionals working with autistic children to be the underlying cause of their problems. In most autistic children, it can be determined that their immune systems are in some way compromised. "Deficiencies in complement (proteins in the blood that destroy foreign cells), various cells, enzymes, and other parts of the immune system are common. It appears that the whole of the immune system in children and adults with autism is out of balance"[35.] It is this underlying decreased immune function that appears to make the child more reactive to anything that taxes his or her immune system. Perhaps further research will be able to determine if the trigger for autistic symptoms is related to any illness, medication, vaccination, or food sensitivity that overtaxes the already compromised immune system of a susceptible child.

Because over 70 percent of the immune system is contained in the bowel, anything that causes inflammation in these tissues also has a profound impact on the immune system. Children with autism commonly suffer from a wide variety of digestive complaints such as chronic diarrhea, constipation, and food intolerances. "Several studies have demonstrated abnormal digestive tract function in autistic children."[36.] As was discussed in chapter two on physiology, there are many of causes of bowel inflammation. Untreated food sensitivities, many medications, absorption of toxins from both outside and within the body, and excessive and prolonged stress are the most common. Anything that causes damage to the bowel wall and makes it leaky can result in symptoms. Children with autism often present with a history of symptoms of food sensitivity and bowel inflammation even as infants. Addressing these issues will improve the function of their immune system.

THE OPIATE-AUTISM CONNECTION

Because children with autism often have bowel inflammation and a decrease in their immune function, they are at risk for an additional concern. In healthy children, the by-products of dairy and gluten based foods move from the small intestine into the large intestine, where the bacteria continue to break them down. They are not absorbed through the bowel wall until they are completely digested. In children with severe food sensitivities or other causes of a leaky bowel wall, it is hypothesized that these particles are permitted to pass through the bowel wall into the bloodstream. This creates an inflammatory response throughout the body and interferes with the nervous system, as well.

Many studies have demonstrated that when gluten and dairy-based foods are not completely digested, they produce by-products that are similar to opiate substances such as heroin and morphine.[37.] These are known as gliadomorphins (from gluten) and caseomorphins (from dairy-containing foods), and they have a significant impact on the nervous system if they are absorbed into the body and travel through the circulation to the brain. Children with autism appear to be increasingly sensitive to this process although the mechanism is still not well understood. This is the reason for the gluten-free, casein-free diet being commonly tried by families with autistic children. "The digestion products of natural foods such as casein and gluten containing grains are able to enter the bloodstream through the leaky bowel wall, where they induce immunological responses and interfere directly with the central nervous system."[38.] Because of the addictive nature produced by these foods, children often crave them and removing them from their diet creates significant resistance. In order to free them from the craving and expand their food choices, gluten and dairy based foods as well as other food intolerances must be removed from their diet 100 percent.

The other type of diet being used for children with autism to address the issue of circulating morphine like substances is the specific carbohydrate diet. It goes one step further than the gluten-free, dairy-free diet and removes all complex carbohydrates. The reason for this is that when bowel inflammation is severe, the small out pouchings called villi in the walls of the small intestine are damaged. These villi contain the enzyme amylase to digest the complex carbohydrates in our diet and they absorb nutrients and allow them to pass into our blood steam to nourish our bodies. The growth, maturation and function of these villi are facilitated by the balance of bacteria in the bowel. Without the enzyme amylase to digest complex starches in the diet, these foods remain undigested in the bowel and ferment. This fermentation releases toxins which further damages the bowel wall and allow food particles such as dairy and gluten to be absorbed without being completely digested.

The specific carbohydrate diet removes all complex starches such as gluten and dairy products but also removes other starchy foods such as potatoes, rice, and other gluten-free grains. (A more comprehensive explanation of this process is contained in chapter two and additional information on these diets can be found in chapter three)

SUCCESSFULLY ADDRESSING FOOD SENSITIVITIES IN AUTISM

While still somewhat controversial in the literature, the impact of diet on the symptoms of autism is widely accepted.[39.] Many children on the autism spectrum have digestive symptoms that impact their quality of life. Whether diet manipulation addresses the symptoms of their autism or whether it simply improves some of their often debilitating bowel issues, it is worth giving a change in diet serious consideration. It is impossible to anticipate the amount of benefit that might be achieved without actually implementing the changes for a month and carefully monitoring the results.

All children—whether facing the challenge of autism or not—are unique. One of the errors that I believe that has been made around the topic of diet and the autism spectrum has been the tendency to believe there is one common cause for symptoms and behaviors in most children. While the gluten-free/dairy-free diet or the specific carbohydrate diets are often attempted by parents, I have also seen children get worse while following one of these plans. They over consume another food that is bothersome to their system and many of their symptoms increase. Families then give up in frustration and the trigger food for their child is missed. The entire idea that food might be at the root of their child's challenges is dismissed and their symptoms continue to worsen over time. I am saddened by this error and hope to encourage people to approach the topic differently.

I believe it is essential to take a complete and accurate history from each and every family. It is not enough to simply assume every child with autism is bothered by dairy, gluten, or complex carbohydrates. It is only by identifying the trigger food unique to each child and then removing it 100 percent for one month that parents can be sure the potential issue of food sensitivities has been addressed. I have many clients for whom the food that was the trigger was an unusual food and would not have been removed from the child's diet by any of the normal elimination diet protocols. Even in those families attempting to follow the specific carbohydrate diet with their autistic child, symptoms many not improve or may even worsen as the child reacts to another food, such as eggs, that is over-consumed on this diet. Again, failure of the diet to work results in families giving up on the entire relationship between food and autism and making what might well be a false assumption.

To determine if your child with autism might benefit from an adjustment in his or her diet, refer to the process to determine the trigger food in chapter three. It is only by removing this food 100 percent from your child's diet for a month and rotating the other things they eat that you will truly know if food is part of the cause of their symptoms.

For children with autism, removing a favorite, over-consumed food may seem impossible. As long as your child remains truly addicted to this food and continues to consume it, they will be resistant to trying any additional foods. While there will be a withdrawal period during which your child's behavior and health may be difficult, once they come through this period, the child will be far more willing to add additional foods to their diet. (Does this seem impossible? I promise you, it is true!) I have witnessed this phenomenon myself in hundreds of my clients. At the beginning of this chapter, the story I shared of a child with autism is true and based on a client of mine who had not spoken for nine years and consumed only plain pasta and pizza with most of the topping scraped off. When we replaced his diet with rice-based pasta and a gluten-free pizza crust, within three weeks, he was speaking in full sentences and eating a much wider variety of foods. This demonstrates clearly the powerful impact of removing the addicted trigger food from this child. He quickly began to consume foods and textures that he had refused his entire life. The impact on the future potential of this child was nothing short of miraculous.

WHERE DO I BEGIN TO CHANGE MY CHILD'S DIET?

Stories like Jason's at the beginning of this chapter are, unfortunately, far too common. According to Autism Canada, "The current statistics suggest that autism is on the rise and affects about one in 165 children in Canada and one in 150 in the United States. It is now recognized as the most common neurological disorder affecting children and one of the most common developmental disabilities."[40.] The number of families struggling to find answers to the challenges they face while balancing this with all their other priorities is also increasing. Autism is a disease that impacts an entire family and taxes both its emotional and financial resources.

Many people with autistic children approach me looking for support to change their children's diets, but truthfully, their lives are already so overwhelmingly busy, they simply can't find the time or energy to do it. My approach is always to spend some time with them first to determine their priorities and to help them clarify which of the therapies they are currently doing are making a significant difference. It is common for these parents to feel that they should try every therapy possible—and in doing so, they create unbelievable stress, both for themselves and their children. I am always amazed how, when I ask parents to share with me which of the multitude of therapies they are doing are the two or three that are actually working, they are always able to name them without a moment's hesitation. Their hearts and heads know what to do, but they fall into the trap of doing more for fear they will be judged as not caring or doing enough.

Information on the process for identification of the trigger food unique to your child can be found in chapter three and the comprehensive signs and symptoms list is found in chapter one. If you take the time to complete both of these forms, you will be able to accurately decide whether or not food is a potential cause of your child's symptoms. A more complete list of topics and issues related to the balance and priorities of your life can be found in chapter five. There are questions in that section to help you identify the places where you would benefit from adjusting some of the areas of your life to make room for a change in your child's diet.

Questions:

What places in your life are successfully offering support to the members of your family as you care for your child with autism?

What areas of your life feel out of balance, overwhelming, exhausting and are draining your energy? What concrete step could you take to begin to decrease this impact?

What type of therapy is your child involved in that you believe is really making a difference? What improvement do you think it is creating?

Take a few minutes to notice if there are other therapies or programs your child or you are involved in that are draining your time and energy and offering only minimal support. What step could you take to let go of some of these?

As you consider the idea of addressing the diet of your child with autism, what challenges do you anticipate? What strategies do you need to employ to address these issues and allow you to find the time and energy to make this change?

FOOD SENSITIVITIES AND CHILDREN WITH OTHER DISABILITIES

One of the most dramatic experiences I have had with children and food sensitivities was my connection with a young boy with a severe facial deformity. He was fed through a tube directly into his stomach because he couldn't swallow. As soon as the care worker at his school where I met him connected his tube and poured in the Ensure, his nose began to run like a tap. The worker told me that this was a common occurrence and that the boy also suffered from multiple ear infections and digestive disturbances. The dairy-based Ensure was the only food he consumed, and it was playing havoc with the rest of his body. His disability was challenging enough, but his diet was making these challenges much greater. His quality of life would be dramatically improved if dairy was removed from his diet and he was fed alternate foods.

In chronic illness of all kinds, it is common for all symptoms that occur to be blamed on the primary disease. Rather that search for other solutions and strategies to address these additional concerns, symptoms are often dismissed or minimized as "just part of the disease". I have repeatedly witnessed tremendous improvements in the symptoms of my patients that have previously been attributed to some other chronic condition. A client of mine, who suffered from Parkinson's disease, found a tremendous improvement in mood and a decrease in his digestive symptoms and pain level when he went on a dairy and gluten-free diet. These symptoms had previously been attributed to his Parkinson's disease. The alleviation of these symptoms has dramatically improved his quality of life.

Many children and adults with disabilities and chronic illnesses also consume a wide variety of medications that can have a significant impact on their digestive tract. If patients take multiple doses of antibiotics to address infections or regularly consume medications that are irritating to their digestive tract, it is highly likely that they will develop some of the symptoms of food sensitivities. As their digestive tract becomes inflamed and the balance of bacteria in their bowel is altered, their ability to tolerate some foods is compromised. By addressing their diets and identifying the trigger foods, these symptoms can be alleviated with a huge improvement in their quality of life. Again, many symptoms being created by medications can be mistaken as symptoms of their disease and remain untreated.

If you have a child with a disability or illness of any kind, I encourage you to refer to the signs and symptoms list in chapter one to see if any of your child's symptoms are there. Rather than attribute all of your child's challenges to their chronic illness or disability, complete the history form in chapter three to identify the trigger food and then remove it from your child's diet for a month. You likely won't find a cure for your child's primary disease, but you may be able to eliminate some symptoms or behaviors that have been having a significant, negative impact on the quality of life of your child and your family.

Questions:

What specific symptoms did you identify on the signs and symptoms list that are negatively impacting the quality of life for your child?

How would the quality of life for your child or your family be improved if some of these symptoms were eliminated or improved?

Once you have identified the trigger food by completing the questionnaire in chapter three, what support do you need in order to to remove this food for a month?

What areas of your life are draining your energy and time that you need to let go of in order to give the diet a try?

What areas of support do you currently have in your life that will support you to make this change?

CHAPTER 7 HIGHLIGHTS

FOOD SENSITIVITIES AND THE AUTISM SPECTRUM

- There is much conflicting and confusing information about the cause and treatment of autism, which makes it very difficult for parents to decide how to help their child. It does seem to be accepted that these children suffer from depressed immune systems, and anything that improves this supports their health and functioning.
- There are a number of diets tried by parents with autistic children but the results and often inconsistent. The strategies offered in this book support parents to find the specific trigger food for their individual child and to increase their chance of success.
- Most families with autistic children are pushed and pulled in many directions as they try to determine what therapies are best suited to their child. Rather than try and do it all, parents need to be selective in what they do and carefully guard the priorities and stress level of their family.

CAUSES OF AUTISM

- In her book, *Gut and Psychology Syndrome,* Dr. Natasha Campbell-McBride addresses what is believed by many professionals working with autistic children to be the underlying cause of the children's problems. In most autistic children, it can be determined that their immune systems are in some way compromised.
- It is this underlying decreased immune function that makes the child more reactive to anything that taxes their immune system. Because over 70 percent of the immune system is contained in the bowel, anything that causes inflammation in these tissues also has a profound impact on the immune system.

THE OPIATE/AUTISM CONNECTION

- There have been many studies that have demonstrated that incompletely digested gluten and dairy-based foods produce by-products that are structurally similar to opiate substances, such as heroin and morphine.
- When these by-products are absorbed into the body through the leaky bowel wall, they are able to reach the brain and result in neurological symptoms and addiction to these foods.
- Children with autism may react to the large number of these by-products in their brains and develop a wide range of symptoms. The by-products of both dairy and gluten-containing foods can be measured in the urine of children with autism.

SUCCESSFULLY ADDRESSING FOOD SENSITIVITIES IN AUTISM

- Children—whether they have autism or not—are unique, so there is no diet that addresses every child's individual needs.
- Some children who follow the gluten-free and dairy-free diet or the specific carbohydrate diet experience an increase in their symptoms. This is the result of an over consumption of a food that their body does not tolerate.
- Rather than attempt a diet that has been successful for other families, the only way to ensure you identify the trigger food causing symptoms is to follow the process identified in this book.
- Because families with autistic children are often financially and emotionally stretched, it is wise to invest time and money in a diet that has the best chance of success rather than making many attempts at changes that are difficult and offer very little change in the child's symptoms.

- In order to succeed, parents must address their entire lives and consider the stresses and commitments already present in their schedules before they simply add another therapy to their already overwhelming schedules. Chapter five offers a process to do this.

WHERE DO I BEGIN TO CHANGE MY CHILD'S DIET?

- Chapter five is all about life balance, stress, having healthy boundaries, resisting the criticism of others, and silencing the sabotaging voices in your head. Addressing some of these issues before beginning the diet change increases your chance of success.
- Take time to complete the signs and symptoms list in chapter one and see how many of your child's symptoms may actually be the result of something he or she is eating. If you identify a number of symptoms on the list, it is very likely that your child's symptoms will improve dramatically when the trigger food is removed.
- Even if your child's diet is very restrictive and they are very sensitive to textures and tastes, addressing their food sensitivities may result in a huge change. Your child's diet choices will expand, and your child will eat healthy foods he or she once refused once this trigger food is eliminated.

FOOD SENSITIVITIES AND THE CHILD WITH OTHER DISABILITIES

- It is common for children with disabilities to have all their symptoms blamed on their disease. It is important to investigate each symptom your child experiences to ensure it isn't related to another cause. Take time to read the signs and symptoms list in chapter one to see how many of your child's challenges are reflected there.
- Food sensitivities can be both a cause and a result of your child's disease. Some medications your child takes may

be causing inflammation in their bowel, resulting in food sensitivity symptoms. The disease itself may also be made worse by the foods your child is eating, so identifying any trigger foods and removing them from your child's diet can significantly improve his or her quality of life.

CHAPTER EIGHT

QUICK SOLUTIONS TO COMMON SITUATIONS

Dealing with Challenges and Resistance in Yourself and Your Family

1. "I don't have time to do this. I work full-time and care for three young children. My husband travels a lot, and I often resort to fast food just to give my children something quick to eat."

   You are another mother—like the rest of us—doing her best to juggle multiple obligations and commitments. I know your plate is full, and adding one more thing feels unmanageable. Chapter five offers an invitation to look at all the parts of your life in order to help you prioritize. What can you let go of, and what are you saying yes to that is not really what you want? Once you clarify that and find the true reason that will motivate you to improve the health of your child, you will find the time. By planning and cooking ahead, your family will get nutritious meals that are quick and easy. Plus, you will spend far less time nagging your children about their behavior, struggling over lost homework with them, or taking them for repeated doctor's appointments. You might even find time for yourself.

2. "I'm just not a motivated enough person, and I hate change. I can already tell it will be too much work and too difficult."

Change is difficult for us all, and you are not alone in finding it challenging. Chapters four and five address this topic and help you to understand a little better what it is that feels difficult and where you are stumbling. You are a motivated person—you simply haven't figured out what motivates you yet. Read that part of the book, and see what you can learn. When you are motivated and connected to the difference a change will make, it becomes much easier to do.

3. "I hate this and want to quit right now!"

What do you think is really going on? Are you stressed because of the diet or because of something else going on in your life? Has someone whose opinion you value criticized what you are doing, or is your own health struggling at the moment? Is there some particular type of help that you are longing for but for which you have been reluctant to ask?

Once this crisis has passed, take a minute to ponder what you are really feeling. If you are in this negative space now, you may have discovered there is nothing for your child to eat, they are starved, and you don't know what to do. It sounds as though your preplanning has fallen by the wayside, and you are feeling frustrated. Take a quick trip to the grocery store or a quick glance through your cupboards and get creative. Find something fun, different, and easy you can create in five minutes to get you over the hump. It might mean buying an already-roasted chicken. It might mean buying some pasta and a jar of sauce for a quick spaghetti dinner. It might even mean going out to a restaurant that serves foods your kids love. Whatever you do, don't give in or give up! Breathe deeply, choose something easy and fun, and when the kids are in bed, regroup. What exactly is causing your upset? Take stock of what happened, and commit to yourself to plan things a little more in advance!

4. "My son is screaming and refusing to eat what I am cooking. I have tried lots of different foods that he is allowed, and he hates them all."

I am assuming that you are serving your son normal, healthy, age-appropriate food and not liver and onions. It is okay that he has preferences, but you are the parent. Avoid the conflict of forcing him to eat what he doesn't want by simply stating quietly that this is delicious food, and it is what is being served for dinner. If he wants to leave the table, let him go, but don't fall into the temptation of offering him a snack a few minutes later. If he is hungry, offer him the plate of the dinner you offered him before in a very positive and friendly manner. If he complains, empathize with his frustration, and remind him that his dinner is here when he is hungry. Resist the temptation to get into a conflict with him or stray from the diet. This is challenging to do and may result in a few angry meals, but he will quietly begin to eat when he is hungry as long as you leave out healthy, appropriate food for him. Part of your goal is to teach him healthy eating habits, so don't give up. Kids also respond well—whatever their age—if you involve them in meal planning and food choices. Ask their opinions, buy some of the things they ask for if they are appropriate, and enlist their help in the preparation. They are far more likely to eat what you serve if they have had some choice.

5. "My husband keeps taking the kids to get ice cream on the weekend after I have worked hard to keep them dairy—free all week! He doesn't want to cooperate with the diet and refuses to remove the cheese from our fridge."

I hear many stories in which husbands sabotage their wives' efforts, and it is sad. When your kids are in bed, sit down quietly with your husband, and listen to his frustrations and concerns. Very often, husbands feed their children trigger foods because they have issues with the very foods their wives are trying to remove and are craving those foods themselves. By taking the kids along, your husband can satisfy his own craving and say he is just having fun with them. It is certainly best if the whole family gives the diet a try, but if he refuses to cooperate, at least ask him to eat the food away from the house and not give it to the kids. It is also important for him to understand why you are altering the diet. Sit together, and talk about the impact the health symptom or behavior will have on your child's future if it continues. Imagine what your child's life will be like in ten years if the symptom doesn't improve. Imagine what your family life might be like! This may help to increase his motivation to support your efforts. If not, perhaps he needs an opportunity to care for the screaming toddler who is out of control due to the ice cream. Book yourself an appointment at the spa, and leave him all day with the kids! This always works!

6. "There is no way that our child will cooperate with this. He goes to school and to after-school care, and it will be impossible to keep him on the diet."

It sounds like the idea feels totally overwhelming. Almost all the time, it is the parent who struggles with making the diet work, and the child actually enjoys the experience of being special. This topic has become far more mainstream than it ever used to be, so schools and organizations are usually more than willing to cooperate if you give them good information about what to do and provide some extra snacks they can keep in their cupboards for emergency birthday parties, etc. We have four kids who lived and thrived despite diet adjustments, and I know hundreds more who have, as well. You can do it if you are organized. You won't always get it perfect—and life isn't about that, anyway. If you do your best to plan ahead, your child will be grateful for your interest.

7. "My mother keeps coming to the house with foods our kids can't eat and then saying, 'I didn't think a little bit would matter.'"

This is another very common and frustrating story. Yes, a little bit does matter, and she can't do it. How strong are your boundaries? How good are you at offering a firm yet compassionate "no"? Don't give in, and explain calmly that you are trying to do the very best for your kids and would love her support. Give her extra ingredients to keep at her house when she is baking, and give her some recipes, too, if you have to. Sometimes the only thing that works is the tears of her grandchildren when you throw away the ice cream cake she brought. Try not to be confrontational in front of your children. Simply explain that nana is learning about what they can eat and hasn't quite figured it all out yet, but model good boundaries for your kids, as well.

8. "It might be a good idea to give this a try, but I haven't the remotest clue how to begin. I would need some support, and I don't have anyone in my life with any knowledge on diet changes or nutrition."

That's why I wrote this book. There is a section in chapter five that deals directly with asking for and finding adequate support, so I encourage you to take time to read it. You will likely be surprised if you ask around your neighbourhood and friends how many others are either struggling to make the same

225

changes or would love to try diet changes if they had someone to share the journey with. Please check out my website at *www.foodsensitivechildren.com* for additional opportunities for support.

9. "When I fall off the wagon and lose my focus, what quick strategy can I use to get back on? It needs to be easy and motivating! I feel like such a lame mother when I don't follow through on what my kids need."

Parents are quick to beat themselves up for being human! You are doing a great job just by taking the time and effort to change your child's diet. It is clear that you care deeply for your family. The best strategy is planning. If you are stressed, there is no food in the house, and the kids are hungry, the situation offers a welcome invitation to cheat. Try keeping a special cupboard with all the ingredients for a few quick and easy meals stocked all the time. Even when the rest of the kitchen is empty, there will be something safe to eat. Also, when you feel the urge to quit and feel your focus fading, stop and notice what it is you are really feeling. Chances are, you are angry about something else in your life, or someone has just stepped boldly over your boundaries. We all have habitual responses that we resort to when we are stressed, and they often are connected to food. It is easier to acknowledge what you are feeling and notice the message your body is offering than to resort to a temporary fix of a food to numb the feeling away. It often helps, as well, to simply get out of the house. Pick up your kids and do something fun, go to a restaurant with safe food, visit a friend, or do something to simply change the energy of your frustration so you can begin again.

10. "My kids are difficult! They never seem to listen or do what I ask, and I am exhausted by the end of the day. I couldn't possibly take on one more thing, and they won't cooperate, anyway."

Your life sounds very stressful and busy. Parenthood can definitely feel overwhelming sometimes. Are you spending more time than you would like nagging your kids and criticizing their behavior? Are you trying your best to get them to take responsibility for some of their things, but they don't seem to get it? What would you think if I offered you the alternative of spending a little more time making muffins and cookies instead of harping at your kids? If you changed their diets and their behavior improved dramatically, what would your life be like then? This isn't a fantasy or an impossible dream, but a very real goal when you find the trigger food. Work your way through the parts of this book that help you find the trigger food and support you to balance your busy life and the give it a whirl. Your family might just be transformed, as mine was.

11. "I am trying to be supportive of my daughter around changing her diet, but she doesn't feel encouraged. She says I am nagging and controlling and that she hates the whole thing. This diet doesn't seem worth harming my relationship with her, even if she is feeling physically better."

Parenting is a challenge at the best of times, as we often try to be supportive—but instead, our kids hear criticism and complaints. You are absolutely right to focus on the relationship you have with your daughter as being what is most important. The short answer is that she is likely at an age where she wants her independence and is pushing back at you because she doesn't feel she has enough choices. Spend some time with her, acknowledge this need, and help her develop a plan that feels more like her own. Ask her what she wants your role to be in this story and how you can best support her. The more you can involve her in the process, the easier it will be. Your job is primarily to ensure that there are lots of healthy and delicious foods for her to eat and pack in her lunches.

However, you are the parent, so don't hear in my comment that you should let her make all the decisions. Just as you did when she was a toddler, offer parameters within which she can choose, and be clear that cheating is not one of them. It is your job as a parent to hold the bar at the place that serves her long-term good—a place she likely doesn't have much ability to see at the moment.

12. "I do a pretty good job most days, but there are certain situations in which I always give in. When I am over-tired or stressed, my child's whining and complaining gets to me, and I usually give her what she wants. What can I do in these situations to help myself stay true to what I really want?"

Can you recognize the voice of your saboteur? This is the internal voice we all have that makes us doubt our decisions and give in to outside pressure, even when we know what is right for us. Take a few minutes to complete the section in chapter five on the voice of your saboteur, and clarify what this voice is telling you. Being aware of what is going on is the first step toward changing it. This voice most often is connected to some old and difficult story that we tell ourselves, so take time to complete that section and clarify what the story is. In the moment, however, the best strategy is to stop. Stop talking. Ask your child to stop talking, and simply disconnect from the situation. Having an agreement with your kids that you never say yes when they whine will decrease this behavior dramatically. When they whine, point it out to them, and disconnect from it. Don't talk about the issue anymore until they can speak in a normal, rational voice. Acknowledge their frustration and anger, but don't get sucked into the story. When you are both calmer, have a conversation about what the real issue is, and come up with a reasonable solution. This strategy works well with kids of all ages and is best begun when your child is a toddler. The more you acknowledge and engage in whining and tantrums, the more your children will use them to get what they want. Life can get very challenging if you have several whiny and belligerent teenagers, so discourage the behavior before you get there.

13. "The rest of my extended family all are late-bloomers and have loads of allergies. I think it is just our family's lousy genes."

You are likely right, but not in the way that you think. Your family probably does share common genes that are causing the sensitivities, but you are not doomed to simply tolerate and live out this perpetual story. When you find the trigger food and remove it, many of the symptoms will disappear. You might just be the catalyst for your entire family finding a renewed sense of health.

14. "*Help!* My son has only eaten four foods for the last year and he refuses to try anything new."

This is another common story! If you have just begun to change your child's diet, this isn't unusual, as he likely gravitated to the few foods that he craved. It usually takes about a week for any withdrawal symptoms to disappear and for the child to become more willing to eat new and different foods. This happens all the time so try your best to wait it out.

When you change the diet, enlist his cooperation and ideas in planning your meals. Teach him how to choose a variety of foods and how he must eat at least three different food groups (or colours, if he is young) at each meal. Also ensure that he has a source of protein at every meal to keep him going in his busy life. Don't allow mealtime to become a struggle, as you won't win! Place his dinner on the table, and if he complains and refuses to eat, just tell him he must stay at the table until everyone is finished, whether he chooses to eat or not. Don't engage in conversation on the topic. Focus on other topics, and allow him to simply leave the table when you are all done.

229

Remind him that his dinner is in the fridge in case he is hungry later on. Above all, resist the temptation to offer him a sandwich or some cereal later on. Who wouldn't choose peanut butter and honey over broccoli and chicken? He will get the message and will eat the food that you prepare. His food choices will expand naturally once the trigger food is removed.

15. "My child has been off the trigger food for three months and seems to be doing well. Can't I try giving her a little bit now to test what happens?"

It depends on many different things. If her symptoms were very mild before and they cleared up quickly, perhaps a *tiny* taste might be okay. Do not give her a lot, and do not let her have it several days in a row when you don't think any symptoms occur. The effect can be cumulative. With food intolerances, the amount she eats is important, so resist the temptation to add the food back every day. If your child's symptoms were severe and you have removed a trigger food, three months is not enough. For example, dairy products should be removed from the diet of a child for one full year before being challenged again. We want the body to have time to heal. If you try it, remember that your child may have a more dramatic response now that her body is beginning to heal, so her symptoms might be more severe. Also, be careful not to add the food back when she is overtired, unwell, or under a lot of stress as this increases the likelihood of a reaction. Be honest with yourself about your reason for wanting to add the food back. Is your child missing the food or is it you that wants to eat it? Has your child's health or behavior improved a great deal and is it worth the risk of adding it back so soon?

16. "My son only eats foods that contain dairy. If I remove those, he will starve!"

Both dairy and gluten-containing foods commonly create this addictive tendency. When they are not completely digested because of inflammation in the digestive tract, the breakdown products are related to opiate-containing drugs, like morphine and heroin. This is partially what accounts for children's natural tendencies to eat more and more dairy to the exclusion of other foods. One of the most dramatic examples I have ever seen of this was when I was watching a TV documentary on addicts in the downtown east side of Vancouver. This courageous woman shared her story, and at the end, asked if she could have her reward. The announcer gave her a platter-sized plate piled at least six inches high with whip cream. She sprinkled dozens of packages of sugar on the top and proceeded to eat it with a spoon. She got a fix from eating the whip cream.

As you remove dairy products from your son's diet, there are a few things to consider. First, plan ahead, and be sure you have loads of healthy and appealing alternatives. Second, part of his craving will be satisfied by having foods of similar textures to the dairy foods he loved, so buy some delicious soya, rice, or coconut ice cream as well as some soya yogurt. The best cheese substitute that doesn't contain casein is made by a company called Daiya foods, and information on their products can be found on the website at *www.daiyafoods.com* Thirdly, keep your child's blood sugar even by offering him small bits of food throughout the day, and be sure each snack has a little protein with it. Protein and fat help to slow the release of the sugars in food and will help his blood sugar to stay more even. And lastly, don't give in. When he craves his old foods, empathize with his frustration, and then offer him a delicious, dairy-free cookie or muffin. Once he has been on the diet for a couple of weeks, his craving will begin to disappear, and he will be willing to eat a wider variety of foods.

17. "My daughter is a very busy and physical five-year-old. I always thought it was just who she was, but now the teachers are

concerned in kindergarten that she is bothering the other kids. Changing her diet won't actually make a difference, will it?"

Diet has a huge impact on behavior. The most dramatic example I have seen is a young girl in kindergarten who was a bully. She kicked over the block castles other kids built, pushed kids off the tire swing, and gave them a shove when they weren't ready at the top of the slide. She had no friends and was not invited for play dates or birthday parties. When we investigated her diet, she ate nothing but chicken—chicken nuggets, chicken burgers, and chicken noodle soup. When we removed the chicken, her behavior was transformed. She stopped being a bully for the first time in her young life and was calm and quiet. She maintained her zest for life and her physical gifts, but no longer aggressively bothered the other kids. Her future potential had been changed by the simple elimination of a trigger food.

Does this sound like your child? Has she always been a bit pushy and aggressive? What do you think will be in her future if this behavior continues? I would encourage you to complete the section in chapter three on finding the trigger food and give it a try. Perhaps your story will be as transforming as the one I just shared.

18. "My child gets sick quite a bit with colds and the flu, but so do all of her friends. Isn't this normal for kids when they are constantly in school with lots of other kids? What is normal, and how do I identify a problem that diet change will help?"

This is a common argument against trying the diet. Yes, it is true that all children get sick and that this is part of building a strong immune system. However, if your child has a perpetual runny nose that most often leads to ear infections, bronchitis, or asthma attacks, this is not normal. Children, if they are healthy, recover from illnesses and return to good health in a few days. If your child is always sick with one bug or another, this is good reason to consider looking for and removing a trigger food. As a mother, I know how difficult it is to be constantly going from one doctor's appointment to another and forever having your children up all night with a cough, an asthma attack, or diarrhea. It is exhausting for everyone involved. My answer to people who resist this idea is that there is nothing harmful about removing a food from a child's diet for a month. There are healthy alternatives for any food that might be removed. It is definitely worth giving it a try.

19. "My ten year old son is cheating on his diet at school. He doesn't confess to doing it, but I can tell by his behavior and symptoms. What do I do?"

This is challenging as kids gets older because we want them to learn to make their own choices and then learn from the consequences. However, there are a few things you can do. First, talk to your son, and listen deeply to his frustrations with the diet. Help your son explore alternative solutions that seem to feel easier. Talk to him about the long-term implications of his symptoms, and look for a reason that is highly motivating to him. If your son knows that his acne will improve or his unpleasant gas will be eliminated, he will be far more likely to cooperate! In the end, you are still the parent. If he continues to make inappropriate choices that impact his health and behavior along with the rest of the family, create a consequence that will matter to him, and then be consistent.

20. "I'll start it after Christmas/after Easter/when he is three/when school is over. Now isn't the right time."

How will you know when the right time is? What is causing you to procrastinate? What price is your child paying while you wait? Chapters four and five in this book will help you evaluate why you are resistant and what parts of your life you might need to address before you will embrace the idea. Take some time to get organized, and complete the questionnaire in chapter three to figure out the offending food. Buy the groceries. Educate your friends and family, and give it whirl. Your child is counting on you to keep his or her best interests at the forefront of your mind and to courageously step up when you need to. There are no more excuses. Figure out what will motivate you to do it, and then get on with it! No time will be perfect, so pick the time during which the withdrawal symptoms will cause the least upset, and start.

21. "If I don't get new ideas for recipes that work and that my kids like, there is no way I can continue this diet! My kids won't eat what I am making, and I am wasting too much food."

Do your best to make delicious and healthy food for your kids, and expect them to eat it. Make the old standbys and comfort food they love with alternative ingredients, as they are more likely to eat those. If you include them in menu planning and preparation, younger kids are also more likely to eat what you have prepared. Be careful not to turn yourself into a short-order cook and try and accommodate the varied tastes of everyone in your family. Simply offer everyone dinner, and if they don't want to eat it, they can sit until everyone is finished and then leave the table. Place their dinners in the fridge, and invite them to eat if they get hungry. Resist the temptation to give them snacks a few minutes later. Their tastes will change once the trigger food has been removed, and they will embrace the new foods if you are patient.

Cooking with alternative ingredients is different and can often be frustrating. I suggest you use the alternatives listed at the back of this book and check out some of the recipe resources I have listed. You can also search the Internet for what you are looking for, as there are loads of amazing websites devoted exclusively to people making a wide variety of diet changes.

22. "My daughter seems to conveniently 'forget' to ask what ingredients are in foods, and this results in her often coming home from a friend's house with a stomach-ache. It keeps sabotaging all the efforts I am making at home. What can I do to help her understand how important it is to eat the correct foods?"

It is a delicate balance in parenting to encourage kids to make independent decisions and yet prevent them from making unhealthy choices. Depending on the age of your child, she will have different opportunities for independent choices. Whatever her age, however, it is important to help her connect to what would motivate her to make the healthy choices her own body needs. None of us make decisions to stick to something we don't want to do and don't believe is worth doing at all. Take a look at the values exercise in chapter five of this book, and spend some time with your child talking about why she should bother doing the diet. What symptoms does she have that are getting in the way of her life? What does she think the long-term impact of these might be if they get worse as she gets older? Where has she been successful in making other good choices for herself, despite peer pressure? What would motivate her to embrace the idea for a month rather than commit to it for a lifetime? Try to get her to find some tangible and meaningful reason to make healthy choices.

Once you have found a compelling reason, help her role-play ways to tell her friends. Come up with clever responses that lighten the topic. Help her also to figure out places she can go to eat that will minimize her experience of feeling different when she is out with her friends, but don't let yourself cave in to her demands. Be clear that you want her to be as healthy as possible and set limits for what you will allow.

23. "What are some fun and quick answers my kids can use when people ask why they can't eat bread? Rather than make it such

a serious topic for them, I'd love them to be able to answer with a clever response. I want them to learn early in life how to counter the resistance and criticisms of others"

It is great to lighten the topic and encourage kids to play with some interesting answers. What they say depends partially on the age of the child. I have heard toddlers announce proudly, "I get a sore tummy" when someone asks why they can't eat the cookie, and I have heard older kids simply say they don't like bread at all. Arm your kids with enough factual information to allow them to be honest. If they have celiac disease, be sure they know the correct name and what it means. The most important part of their answers is the energy with which they say them. I love how toddlers and school-age kids often embrace the diet changes as it makes them feel special and they are proud to announce, "I can't eat pizza, so I get a bag of gummies instead!" Even teenagers can answer in a very matter-of-fact way that they get really sick when they eat it, and it just isn't worth it. If your kids have been raised with a matter-of-fact attitude around the topic, they won't offer any drama when they talk about it in their lives. It is just like wearing braces or glasses and is simply part of who they are. If you treat the issue this way at home, your kids won't shy away from comments about it. They might also educate their peers a little because you can bet many of them are experiencing the same challenges. I love the comments sometimes made by teenage boys on the topic of their symptoms. Sometimes their goal is to gross the other person out with a graphic description! It usually gets a huge laugh, and their friends certainly help their friend eat well because the consequences sound awful, and they don't want to be around if something bad happens.

24. "I am getting angry with my kids more than I ever used to. I am frustrated with their symptoms, yet I am finding this diet is consuming my waking thoughts and life. I go to lots of trouble

to make delicious food, and then they complain or won't eat it. I just blow up!"

Spending lots of time and energy—never mind money—on diet changes for the health of your kids and meeting nothing but resistance is stressful and irritating! You are not alone nor unique in your experience. Perhaps there is simply too much on your plate, and the diet was the last piece to tip you over. I suggest you look at the section in chapter five on balancing your busy life, and notice how much you are trying to do. Can you say no to the things that drain your energy? Are you choosing for yourself how your day unfolds, or are you wedging your priorities around everyone else's needs? What important value of yours are you stepping right over? What meaningful choices are you longing to make that don't seem to fit on your calendar? You are the captain of your own ship, so decide what is important, and sail in that direction. Don't let the hot air of other's expectations determine what you do. Create space in your life for what matters, and get rid of the things that don't. You will feel less stressed and overwhelmed and will enjoy your kids and your life more.

Removing a much-loved food from the family diet results in feelings of loss and anger is one of the normal stages everyone experiences. All those fun visits to Dairy Queen! Family pizza night! Birthday cheesecakes! What a shame they are gone! Allow yourself space to grieve for the things that have been lost, and then turn your focus to creating new rituals for your family. Go to a new ice cream store and have a sorbet! Have Chinese food instead of pizza! Make a soy cream cheese birthday cake instead! As you grieve the changes and find new solutions, your frustration with it all will decrease. You will find your way; it just takes a little time. There is a section in chapter four that deals with the feelings of grief and loss related to diet change so perhaps reading that will help you recognize that the anger you are experiencing is normal.

25. "It might be possible to do this diet with an infant or a toddler, but I can't imagine for a minute that my older child or teenager will cooperate with it. What is the point in starting something my child will likely abandon when he is older?"

This is a question that could be answered with an entire book of reasons. First, the health of your child as an adult depends very much on the diet and lifestyle he has when he is young. There is very compelling research that shows that childhood obesity predisposes kids to many challenges as adults. The same is true for food reactions. I see many adults who have long and difficult stories of health, behavior, and learning challenges all through their lives. Many of these could have been avoided if their diets had been adjusted in childhood.

Often, it is the parents that struggle with the diet, and not the kids. Kids actually like to feel well and be active in their lives. They don't like to feel awful, have offensive gas, get sick all the time, struggle in school, or have no friends, so they are often very motivated to do anything that helps. Don't sell your child short on what you think they can or will do. Kids are remarkably resilient and will do lots of things if they are motivated and believe they make a difference in their lives. The extra benefit of teaching your child to stand up for what is right for himself is that he will have lots of practice saying no. He will be better prepared to say no to peer pressure in his teenage years.

26. "I am lost in figuring out what food is the culprit for our son. I have narrowed it down to about four, but I can't figure out which food it is. There is no way I am doing all four!"

One of the reasons why my approach to food sensitivities is different is because of my belief in the concept of trigger foods. For twenty-seven years, people have come to see me with long lists of foods they have been asked to remove by another health care professional, and they are overwhelmed. Sometimes the list contains over twenty foods! Chapter three is devoted to helping you find the most likely trigger food, so take time to read it. The short answer is that the food that is usually an issue is the one that is eaten almost every day, craved in some form or another, reached for when your son is stressed and overtired, bothersome to other people in your family, and the one your son would be most reluctant to give up! When you ask yourself these questions, I am confident you will find your answer. Once you have identified the trigger food, remove it 100 per cent for a month and see what happens. You will find support to do this successfully in the other chapters of this book.

27. "I am angry about having to do this! My friend's kids seem to eat nothing but pizza and spaghetti and never have tummy aches or ear infections. Why me and my kids?"

It's irritating, isn't it? There are kids—and even entire families—who seem able to eat whatever they want and never get sick. They are, however, very rare—and certainly rarer than you think. Over the years, I've seen firsthand how often people hide the challenges they are experiencing at home. While their children appeared to have it all together at school, they were often struggling with some issue at home. More than a few of them were still wetting their beds at the age of ten or taking medications to help them deal with behavior issues. I know that on the days when the diet seems too much and you long to just go and pick up a pizza like other people can do, it is difficult. I acknowledge the efforts you are taking and can assure you that you are making a dramatic difference in your child's life. My children have been eating this way for over twenty-five years, and my husband and I have reaped the benefits of all our effort. The symptoms and issues of their childhoods are gone, and each of them is an amazingly healthy, strong, fit, and successful adult. I know as a mother that would not be the case had we not addressed their issues when they were young. It is, in fact, one of the reasons I wrote this book and why I love the word hope. It is amazing to watch your child grow, thrive, and become exactly who there were created to be. Celebrate your courage in making the sometimes difficult choices, and trust that you and your child will be grateful for what you have done down the road.

28. "The rest of my family has all the same symptoms as we have, and no one else will pay attention to them or even give the diet a try. They load themselves up with pills and then continue to complain about how unwell they all feel. If they would only give the diet a try, I know it would help. Why won't they listen?"

This is the same story as the question above, and the same answer applies. Lead by example, and demonstrate how much improvement you have seen in your family's health and behavior since removing the trigger food. As you enlist their support to create appropriate food at family potlucks, they will begin to see that it is possible to eat delicious yet healthy food. Resist the temptation to push people into changing, as they will only change when they are motivated internally. You can, however, cultivate this a little by encouraging them in places where you know they will be motivated. For example, if your teenage sister has bad acne, helping her see that removing dairy from her diet might improve it may encourage her to try it.

Special Occasion Strategies

1. "My son has been invited to a birthday party, and they are having pizza and an ice cream cake! He is on a dairy-free diet! What on earth can I do?"

First of all, whatever the age of your child, ask him what he wants to do. Don't assume that you know. If your child is a toddler or school-age, he will most likely be agreeable if you bring an alternate food. Make homemade pizza with a topping made from a dairy-free cheese, or simply cover it with his favorite topping, and leave the cheese off. You can buy premade pizza crusts or make your own. For the ice cream cake, either create your own, or allow your child to simply say, "No thank you." To make an ice cream cake, simply allow a dairy-free ice cream to melt slightly, press it into a spring form pan, and refreeze it. When frozen, allow him to decorate it with dairy-free candies and drizzle dairy-free chocolate sauce over the top. It is fun for him to do it with you. You can also simply bake some appropriate cupcakes and have your child take them along. If they don't want to be different, just feed him before he goes, and he can eat only chips and pop. This is a great treat in itself.

2. "I feel mean telling my child he can't participate in pizza day at school. Won't he be harmed by feeling so different or left out?"

It is difficult as parents to watch our children be different, even though we want them to choose what is best for themselves. Be creative in finding a solution, and enlist your child's help. Take him McDonald's or Subway, pack a special treat in his lunch, or allow him to come home. Above all, talk to your child about the experience, but don't place your attitudes on him. He may be just fine with a special treat in his lunch but react to your negative energy on the topic.

3. "Family dinners and celebrations revolve around food at our house. If our diets had to change, so would the menu of these events, and our family would find that very difficult. We even have a family pizza and movie night once a week, so what would we do about that?"

Food does play an important role in family gatherings and everyone looks forward to those old family favorites. Sometimes, it simply isn't possible to make a substitute taste the same. Grieve the loss of this familiar food, and then be creative in replacing it with something else. Most of the time, it is the tradition and company that is important, rather than a specific food. For family movie nights, enlist the kids' ideas of what other foods you might have. You will be amazed how quickly and easily pizza night can become Chinese food or sushi night.

4. "My daughter goes to sleepover birthday parties often, and the food is always pancakes with whip cream, etc. She is nine and finds it difficult to be different. What can I do?"

Little girls love sleepover parties, and it is fun to be invited to go. Talk to the mom ahead of time and determine what the menu is going to be so you can match what is being served. If your child is simply off dairy, offer to buy alternate milk that can used for pancakes, cookies, birthday cakes, etc. If the food is gluten, the challenge is a little greater, and you might need to send along your own premade pancakes or waffles or a mix for her to use. The best alternative, however, is the one your child will cooperate with. Talk to her about her experience, and decide what plan feels best to her. Be clear, however, that eating a trigger food is not an option and that you are counting on her to be honest in what she does. Send along some special treats she can share, and help her focus on the other fun aspects of the birthday party. If the whole idea of a breakfast she can't or won't eat is too difficult, you can certainly go and pick her up before they go to bed and take her home early. Some children actually prefer this option, so be sure you ask.

5. "My daughter is going on dates and doesn't want to be different. What can she do?"

The best policy is honesty. If your child was seriously allergic to peanuts, she would have to tell her date. She can be very casual about it, say she can't eat a particular type of food, and suggest a few places that she can eat. I am always adamant that people not shy away from eating out. It is important to be social, so go out for dinner and simply ask the restaurant to accommodate your needs. Most are very good. I would suggest you encourage your daughter to try and see being different as being unique rather than weird. I know teens like to belong, but a little practice speaking up for herself might just help her say no to sex, drugs, and alcohol when the time comes.

6. "My daughter wants to go to camp with her friends, but I can't imagine how this would be possible and still keep her off milk. If she has milk at camp, it will be a problem for her, as she will develop a stomach-ache again and may even go back to wetting her bed. Is there any way this can work?"

Going away to camp is very possible but requires a little planning. Our four kids all did it often, and in most situations, it worked well. Over the last few years, the awareness of food sensitivities has increased so much that most camps are now very accommodating. Soya milk is commonly provided and even vegetarian and vegan meals are offered. I suggest you contact the camp and speak directly to the cook. Get a sense of what the menu contains, and ask the cook what support you can offer to make it work for them as well as your child. I often sent along a box packed with gluten-free pasta, allowable cookies, and other staples so the camp cooks didn't have to purchase it themselves. I always gave this box to the counsellor myself so our kids could board the bus with the others. The biggest issue, however, is the attitude of the camp. They need to be willing to embrace your child as just a regular kid and to do what they can to minimize the impact of her diet. Talk with them up front about their plan, and emphasize the importance of quietly supporting your child to stay healthy. If they seem totally overwhelmed by the idea and uncooperative, find another camp. The camp our children attended that managed their diets amazingly well was

Educo in 100 Mile House, B.C. Their website is *www.educo.ca/ advenureschool.php*

Dealing with Physical Symptoms

1. "My son has been losing weight since I have changed his diet, and he can't afford that."

   There are many reasons children lose weight. If your child has been underweight for some time, his weight may increase once he has eliminated the trigger food for a month or more. This is common. If your child is simply not eating adequate calories, reassess what you are feeding him. Offer higher-calorie foods like nuts or avocado, but resist the temptation to offer him junk food just because of the calories. If he is not eating his lunch, enlist his support in making it so it contains things he enjoys, and be sure to pack extra food. If your child picks away at mealtime and is hungry in between, leave out small plates of a wide variety of healthy snack foods that are easily accessible to him all day long. If your child's weight continues to decrease, take him to the doctor for a check-up. Remember, as well, that the pediatric growth charts show only average trends in children and each child is an individual. If your child is healthy, growing, and happy, then he is okay.

2. "We have removed the major offending food, and our daughter's symptoms are about 80 percent better. We are grateful for that but are wondering what we can do about the remaining 20 percent, as it is still causing difficult symptoms for her. Don't tell me there is another food we have missed!"

   A couple of things might be going on. First, check that you have read all the labels on your food products carefully and that every trace of the offending food has been eliminated. Even small amounts make a difference. Second, are you rotating the other foods? Often, without realizing it, people replace one over-consumed food with another over-consumed alternative. Children with the potential to develop food sensitivities often develop symptoms if any food is consumed day after day. The most common instance is when parents replace dairy products with soya products. Before they realize it, they are eating soya cheese, soya cream cheese, soya milk, and soya ice cream—and then soya causes a new set of symptoms.

It is easiest to develop a meal plan for your family that is on a two-week or a monthly rotation so you can pay attention to how often you feed them certain foods. Don't gasp at the idea before you give it a try. I found it to be a very successful way of planning ahead. I wasn't always trying to think of new ideas for dinner, as I had taken the time to plan ahead and ensure I had the required groceries. If you have done all of this and the symptom still persists, it is possible that there is a second trigger food. Follow the same process you did to find the initial trigger food, and see if you can figure out what it is. It will be a food that is eaten almost daily and one that your child craves. Remove this food for a month, and see if the last 20 percent of her symptoms disappear. In children who are otherwise healthy and haven't had huge doses of antibiotics or medications, this other food most often improves and is tolerated in small doses occasionally. The main trigger food, I'm afraid to say, rarely disappears enough for the child to have anything more than the occasional nibble, and even that may bring on symptoms.

The other thing to consider is the pace of your child's life. If she is very stressed or over tired, other secondary foods may be a problem. Often a change in routine and a little extra sleep make a big difference.

3. "I have two children, and both of them have bladder symptoms. Our son is nine years old and still wets the bed, and our daughter has recurrent burning around her labia. She also frequently has to run to the bathroom in a hurry and sometimes doesn't make

it. These symptoms are having a dramatic effect on our kids, and they are afraid to go for sleepovers at their friends' houses. My husband also wet the bed at night until he was ten, and the doctor says my son will outgrow it." Is it possible that these symptoms are related to something they are eating?"

This is a common story. Finding the trigger food and removing it should completely eliminate the symptoms of both of your children. This is a perfect example of the social impact of food sensitivities. The most common food for these symptoms is dairy products. Because your husband suffered from similar symptoms, changing your entire family's diet might make some longstanding symptoms of his disappear, as well. Complete the questionnaire in chapter three to identify the trigger food for each of your children as well as your husband and then remove them from your family's diet completely for a month. Be sure to complete the process for each person in case the trigger food is different, although it is very likely several family members are all bothered by the same food.

4. "I am having trouble remembering how things used to be before we changed our family diet. I think our daughter is feeling better, but I didn't really keep track of how often her tummy aches happened, so it is easy to forget. My mother says she is much better, but I'm not really sure."

How lovely, on the one hand, to forget those difficult days. Journaling is the best way to keep track of the symptoms as you adjust your daughter's diet. It is easy to forget how things used to be, and it is also fun to celebrate even the small changes that occur. I often have parents say that even qualities they thought were just part of their children's personalities changed. One child who was never a morning person all of a sudden came skipping down the stairs and appeared in the kitchen with a gleeful "Good morning." His mother almost fell over. I suggest you continue removing the trigger food for a month and then reintroduce it to see what symptoms might reappear. If you have removed a food that was having a dramatic impact on your child, the symptoms will reappear more dramatically when you give her the food again. You will then be able to see if your efforts have been making a difference.

5. "We are doing the diet really well and our son is feeling much better, but now another symptom has appeared."

The likelihood here is that your son has over-consumed some food he has a borderline issue with. Check your child's diet, and look for a food he consumes almost every day. Look for a pattern in your child's symptoms to see if you can notice when the problem appears. It is absolutely essential that you remove the trigger food *and* rotate the other foods your child eats. When a child has a problem with one food, he or she is at much higher risk of developing a problem with another food if it is over-consumed. This doesn't mean your child can't eat it, but they must do so in moderation.

6. "We have been completely free of eggs in our house for a month, and it doesn't seem to have made any difference at all. Is there any point in trying another food, or does this mean that food isn't the reason for our symptoms?"

If you have carefully completed the signs and symptoms list in this book and have ticked off a number of them, the chances are very good that at least some of your symptoms are related to food. Go back and redo the questionnaire in chapter three that helps you identify the trigger food, and see if you can discover another one. I have had people who ignore what the questionnaire says because they simply can't bear the idea of removing the trigger food that was identified. Check in with yourself to see if you might have done this without being consciously aware. Also, be sure you have removed the eggs 100 percent from your diet. Have you read all the labels to ensure egg powder or something else wasn't hidden in a food you have been eating every day?

7. "What are probiotics? If I gave them to my kids, would it enable them to eat the food that bothers them more often?"

Probiotics are simply a way to reintroduce some of the strains of organisms that are often destroyed or out of balance as the result of multiple courses of antibiotics, stress, a diet loaded with junk food, or other foods or substances that cause inflammation in the bowel. They are very useful to help improve digestion once the trigger food or other cause of the bowel inflammation has been removed. Probiotics restore the balance of organisms that perform a number of important functions in the gut. If the cause of the inflammation is not removed, however, no amount of probiotics will help. It is also important to read the ingredients on the probiotics you choose, as many are cultured on dairy and soya and may cause additional symptoms if these foods are poorly tolerated. It is always wise to take probiotics during a course of antibiotics and to continue for an additional two weeks following the last dose to help recolonize the bowel with good bacteria again.

8. "I am confused by my child's symptoms. Sometimes I give him a food, and it bothers him—and other times, it doesn't seem to be a problem."

Food sensitivities are life-related as well as impacted by the amount of a food that is eaten. If you are on holiday in Hawaii and well-rested, you can often get away with eating a small quantity of a food that is an issue at home when life is busier and more stressful. Foods are also more of a problem when eaten in combination with another potentially bothersome food. If your child is bothered by dairy products and slightly by gluten, as well, eating pizza is more likely to cause symptoms than either of the trigger foods if eaten alone. Food sensitivity reactions can also take up to twenty-four or even thirty-six hours to appear, so they can also be easily missed or confused with an illness or a reaction to another food. This is why I recommend searching for the trigger food and removing only that one to start with. In my experience, all the other secondary foods become less bothersome and can be eaten in moderation.

9. "Won't my children's bones crumble without any milk?"

Children need a balance of nutrients, and no one food is more important than another. Certain lobby groups have done a good job of conditioning us to believe that there is one perfect food that we need to eat several times a day. What children really need is a varied and healthy diet. In my experience, many of the children I see are addicted to dairy products and consume them in some form at every meal. It is not unusual for a parent to bring a three-year-old into emergency with asthma whose dietary history shows they only drink milk. When you remove a trigger food, your child will naturally be willing to expand their food choices. They will eat more fruits and vegetables and be willing to try new and unusual foods. If the trigger foods you have removed are dairy products, simply use fortified rice, soya, or almond milk instead, and add lots of other calcium-containing foods to your child's diet. There are also many kid-friendly calcium supplements you can use if you are concerned. Supporting your child to have a physically active lifestyle also facilitates bone growth and decreases their risk of developing osteoporosis as an adult.

10. "My child is allergic to oranges and gets eczema every Christmas when the mandarin oranges come out. I give her an antihistamine, but it never helps. Perhaps it isn't really oranges at all, and I shouldn't bother taking her off them."

Most food reactions are intolerances and not true allergies. With intolerances, there is no production of histamine, and thus antihistamines don't offer any relief. It is entirely possible that your child is sensitive to oranges and that the extra consumption of them over Christmas along with the busy pace of the holiday season has simply tipped her over the edge. Her sensitivity may be such that during the rest of the year, an occasional orange might not cause symptoms, but you won't know until you give it a try.

11. "We are doing okay on the gluten-free diet, and our son loves all the gluten-free cookies, cakes, etc., but he seems more tired now than he was before we changed his diet. Do you have any thoughts on why this might be?"

When gluten is removed from a child's diet, he often craves the breads, cakes, and cookies he used to have. It is very helpful to replace them initially with tasty alternatives, but eventually you need to shift your child's diet to healthier substitutes. Baked goods are great as a treat and as incentives to stay on the diet, but the focus of his meals and snacks should be on fruits, vegetables, nuts, and healthy gluten-free bread. If your child is eating a diet that contains lots of gluten-free baked goods with sugar, he may not be getting adequate nutrients to support healthy growth and activity. I encourage everyone to ensure that their child has three food groups at every meal or snack—a source of protein, a starch carbohydrate, and a fruit or vegetable. If you vary the things you offer, your child should have all the nutrients he needs, and his energy should return.

12. "I think my son's very busy behavior is just how he is. It might be challenging, but I don't think it is related to food. My husband was like this as a child, as well, and he has turned out fine."

Kids have a wonderful variety of personalities, and we want to embrace them just as they are. The line is crossed, however, when a child's behavior begins to have a negative impact on his self-esteem. If he is constantly being corrected and disciplined or is isolated or ostracized by his peers, it is worth considering adjusting his diet. The goal of diet adjustment—as well as the many other interventions you can try—is to maximize the potential of your child and not to make him into something he is not. On your part, there must be a readiness to change. If you aren't connected to some significant reason for doing it, you will not be successful but will continually sabotage your own efforts and the efforts of your child. It is also possible that if you change your family's diet, your husband will also discover that a food was the cause of his own lifelong issues.

13. "Why are so many kids now being diagnosed with food sensitivities? My parents and my generation seemed to be able to eat anything, and now my kids have all these sensitivities."

It is true that many food-related illnesses are on the rise. Asthma is increasing at a frightening rate, and autism now affects almost one in 100 kids. (see chapter seven for additional information.) There are a number of factors involved here. First, our food supply is now grown in places where loads of pesticides are used, and hormones and drugs are commonly fed to the animals. These substances appear in the foods that we eat and were never part of the diet of previous generations. Also, more and more fast food is available, and more families make a habit of regularly eating highly processed food. In previous generations, mothers were often home and had time to create their meals from scratch. Taking the time to create healthy, nutritious meals that are free of chemicals, pesticides, and unhealthy fats will dramatically improve the health of our next generation of children.

There has also been a tremendous increase in the awareness of food sensitivities and the symptoms they can create. Many children in the past suffered and even died from diseases like asthma, and many left school because of severe learning disabilities that went unsupported. Now more and more children are getting help for these symptoms. Unfortunately, however, food is still not well recognized as a valid cause or contributing factor of many childhood illnesses and there is more work to be done to disseminate this information

14. "I tried removing milk from our son's diet a few months ago, and it didn't make any difference. His symptoms remained exactly the same."

Your story is common and another reason I wrote this book. Unless you read all the labels and knew what you were looking for, chances are that you missed the milk in quite a few places. It hides in unusual foods and is called by numerous names, so it is difficult to remove it all unless you know what to look for. Refer to the list of words indicating dairy in a food in chapter six. In order to decide if the food is the cause of the symptoms, you need to remove it 100 percent for an entire month. Nothing less will give you the correct information. Because you tried it once, I imagine you must be suspicious about the milk in your child's diet, so I encourage you to use this book, and try it again. There is also a possibility that you removed the wrong food and that dairy is not actually the trigger food causing all the symptoms. Only by completing the questionnaire in chapter three and signs and symptoms form in chapter one in this book can you be sure that you are removing the correct food.

15. "I think both our kids and I are bothered by bread. It is in almost every meal that we have, and we all *love* fresh buns and bread. I am afraid I will have withdrawal symptoms when I remove it, so should I remove it from all of us at the same time, or should I consider changing my own diet first?"

This is a great question, and the answer depends on what works best for you. Some moms choose to change their own diets first so they can figure out how to do it as well as go through their own withdrawals first. If you anticipate your withdrawal symptoms might be a challenge, I suggest you do yourself first or last, but not at the same time as you are trying to cope with your withdrawing kids. If your fuse is short and your temper is quick, the experience will be more difficult for everyone.

16. "How can I distinguish a symptom from things that are simply part of my child's personality or a normal stage of development?"

This is a great question. I am a mother of four grown children, and I understand the challenge of parenthood. I would *never* suggest that you embark on a diet or do anything else that has the sole purpose of moulding your child into something he or she is not. My rule of thumb here is that if your child has a health challenge, behavior, or learning issue that is having a negative impact on their life or will likely do so in the future, it deserves to be addressed. Have you ever had your child home sick with the flu for a few days and discovered a loving, warm, affectionate little child who you rarely see sitting on your lap? Wouldn't you love that experience a little more often? I hear this story a lot and have experienced it myself. When your child has the flu and isn't able to eat for a few days, some of the symptoms of their food sensitivity disappear. The child you are holding on your lap is your real child—the one who, despite having a fever or a cold, is calm and peaceful. Children have a wide range of natural gifts and personalities, but often their health, their diets, their life circumstances, and other things get in the way. If your child is struggling in their life, you can do something to help. Listen. Empathize. Take action, and help change your child's story. Their self-esteem is their most prized possession, so help your child be who they are meant to be by finding answers to their struggles. The child who will appear will be the one you knew was there all along!

I have personal experience with this story. One of our children was very unwell, irritable, confused, angry, and difficult. When

I changed the diet, all these symptoms disappeared in two weeks. The teacher at preschool phoned and wanted to know what I had done to my child, who was alert, bright, interested, interactive, and cooperative. It was a life changing experience for both my daughter and me so I encourage you to embrace the idea and try it for yourself.

17. "My daughter has been on the diet for six months and was doing really well until two weeks ago. All of a sudden she has broken out in hives and the antihistamines the doctor prescribed are not helping much at all. She is miserable and unable to go to school and I haven't any idea what to do. The doctor says he may need to try prednisone if it doesn't get better. We have also searched our home for anything new we have used such as soaps, detergent etc and can't find a thing."

Your story is not unusual and it has an easy solution. What has likely happened is that as you have altered the diet of your family and added more healthy foods such as fish, berries, avocado, and tomatoes, the number of foods that contain histamine has dramatically increased. We all have a threshold for histamine that we inherit and when this level is surpassed, we experience symptoms. Hives that result from histamine intolerance do not respond as well to antihistamines such as Benadryl as do hives related to a true food allergy such as peanuts or strawberries. The solution to your daughter's symptoms is to temporarily remove all the foods in her diet that contain histamine. Please see Dr. Janice Joneja's website at *www.allergynutrition.com* for a complete list. Once you have done this, you can begin to taper off any antihistamines that she is taking and see if her symptoms have disappeared. It would also be helpful to add some probiotics to her diet to help restore the balance of bacteria in her bowel. Some of these bacteria produce histamine and this will add to her total histamine load. Because histamine intolerance is related to a level of histamine, your daughter may be able to eat some of these foods in isolation as long as she doesn't eat too many of them at once. Please also check out the website *www. histame.com* for information on an enzyme that she can take that will help to break down histamine in the body. This enzyme is taken fifteen minutes before eating and often dramatically increases tolerance to high histamine foods. In chapter three you will find a more extensive explanation about histamine intolerance.

It is also wise to create a plan to rotate the foods your family is eating. I suggest you create a spreadsheet or chart where you use different meats, fruits, vegetables, grains, legumes and spices each day of the week. Aim to develop a plan where no single food is eaten more often that every four days. This makes meal planning easier and avoids over consumption of any one food. Please check out my website at *www.foodsensitivechildren.com* for a sample rotation menu.

Coping with Resistance from Friends, Coworkers, Teachers and Health Care Professionals

1. "My family doctor does not support my efforts in changing my child's diet, as he says it is unproven that food has any impact on physical diseases, such as asthma."

   I hear this story all the time! This book contains many medical and scientific references that address this issue. I have great empathy for parents who find themselves in this difficult dilemma. You know your child best, so collect the best information you can, and then choose what seems right. Removing a food from a child's diet does not harm the child as long as you replace that food with healthy alternatives. Depending on the age of your child, replace the milk with a fortified soya, rice, or almond milk, and add liquid or chewable calcium to his or her diet. Your child's bones won't crumble, and their asthma might well improve! I have cared for many children whose asthma has dramatically improved, so I encourage you to give it a try.

2. "The allergist says our daughter is not allergic to milk. Her scratch test was normal, yet she continues to vomit and get a runny nose every time she eats something with dairy. I think she should come off dairy, but the allergist doesn't agree. What is going on?"

Take a few minutes to read chapter two on the differences between food allergies and intolerances. The test your doctor used is very accurate for true allergies, but most food reactions are intolerances. The difference is that in food intolerances, there is no release of histamine; thus, no little bump appears on the area that has been scratched. The only sure way to know if a food is causing a reaction is to remove it 100 percent for a month and see what happens. Just because a scratch test is normal does not mean that a child isn't bothered by the food. Take a few minutes to complete the section on identifying the trigger food in chapter three, and see what you learn. Remove this food, and see if your daughter's symptoms disappear. A parent's intuition is an important tool, also, so listen to your gut, and give it a try.

3. "The school won't cooperate with me. Kids bring in birthday and holiday treats that I don't know about, and my child comes home really upset."

You need to plan ahead. Send a stash of special cookies, fruit leathers, or something else your child thinks is a very special treat to school, and have the teacher keep them. When an unexpected cake appears, your child can choose one of his or her special treats. Ask the teacher to let the class know about your child's diet, as many parents are more than delighted to be accommodating. On days like Halloween, Christmas, etc., be sure to offer to send delicious and fun treats that your child will be able to eat and will enjoy sharing with their friends.

4. "My son is struggling with reading at school and is now in a special reading group. The school counsellor says he has a

processing disorder and will always struggle and that diet won't make any difference."

Diet has a very significant impact on learning, attention span, and the processing of information. See the reference section at the back of the book for other credible resources on the topic. My answer to many parents such as yourself is, "What do you have to lose by giving it a try?" The potential for improvement is great, and the risk of doing it is almost nothing. If you follow the format in this book and figure out the trigger food, you will have a good sense of where to begin. Imagine the impact on your child's future potential if you could improve his ability to process and retain what he learns. His self-esteem will also soar as he sees himself as capable rather than stupid. I have personally worked with many families where this has been the case.

5. "I am struggling with all the misinformation around me. Doesn't anyone else know that the food you put in your mouth obviously impacts your health and behavior? I have many friends with bratty kids who have constantly running noses, and my friends won't do anything about it! It is driving me crazy to watch, because I care about these people and their kids."

It is difficult to watch, isn't it? I have had the same experience and have learned the hard way it is best to be quiet. I know it is particularly difficult when it is people you care about or people whose situation is causing huge grief either to them or to their children. The best thing you can do is model what you believe as you live it. Don't comment on it, and don't push the topic on other people. When your friends notice how well-behaved your child is, tell them you know your child's diet plays a big part. If they are interested, offer them this book, my website, or invite them to a workshop on the topic of food sensitivities. There are loads of wonderful resources listed at the back of this book. In the end, however, it is best to simply lead by example and hope that they will be so impressed with the health and behavior of your family that they will follow your lead.

6. "My kids go to friends' homes for play dates and continue to come home having eaten something wrong. The mom tried her best but thought a little bit wouldn't matter. She didn't read the labels and didn't realize that some corn chips have milk. What am I supposed to do so my kids can still play with friends without getting sick?"

This is another common challenge as you change your family's diet. The best strategy is always honesty and information. Phone the mom in the evening when she has more time to talk, or invite her over for coffee. Explain your child's needs, and ask her what you can do to make it easy for her. Tell her you love the idea of your kids being friends and want your kids to be able to play there often. Give her some safe cookies to keep in her cupboard as well as a list of snack ideas your child can have. Most healthy snacks, like fruits and veggies, are usually okay and accepted by most moms as the best choices anyway. If she still doesn't cooperate fully, educate your child, and then pack an extra snack with his or her lunch to be eaten in the afternoon. Make sure it is a fun food, and include enough for a friend they can share. In the end, the most important thing is to educate your own children on how to speak up and make good choices for themselves.

7. "My mother-in-law looks after our kids quite a bit, and she *loves* to cook fancy desserts and treats for the kids. I could never tell her she had to stop."

She doesn't have to. By giving her the alternative milk, flour mix, etc. that your child needs, you can support her to keep cooking in a way that reinforces your efforts to make your child well. Talk to her about your reasons for doing it, and help her understand the long-term implications for your children if their health or behavior doesn't improve. When all is said and done, be clear in your boundaries, and stand firm. Don't give in just to be nice. Make it clear that you intend to give this a very conscientious try and would love her support.

Making the Changes Sustainable

1. "The food is too expensive, and we can't afford to keep this diet up."

   The diet initially does seem more expensive as you explore the various alternative foods you can use. My goal in this book is to offer you alternative ingredients that will allow you to simply adapt family favorite foods. Resist buying expensive, premade food, and make your things from scratch whenever you can. Check out the Internet for loads of amazing recipes that address your specific diet needs. Also, don't fall into the trap of letting your kids convince you that they need all those special cookies, treats, etc. Fruits and veggies are still the cheapest and healthiest foods for kids.

2. "What does it really mean to rotate foods? I want to feed my daughter correctly, but I am confused."

   It means that you try as best you can not to offer your daughter a food any more often than every four days. I suggest you buy small quantities of a wide variety of foods. Instead of buying the huge bag of apples, buy four apples, four oranges, four bananas, a mango, a papaya, some grapes, and some strawberries. When one food is gone, she must choose another one. When all the food is gone, you can buy more. Do the same thing with types of cereals, juices, etc. When one type is gone, she knows she must eat the other ones before you buy more. Also, if she is a toddler, tell her that she must have at least three different colours on her plate, and allow your child to choose. This ensures your child gets a balanced diet and learns colours along the way! You can download a copy of a sample, kid friendly rotation diet from my website at *www.foodsensitivechildren.com*

3. "I don't have time to do this."

It sounds like you have a runaway life with too many things on your calendar and not enough time for everything. What is important to you? How do the symptoms your child is experiencing impact your life and your child's life? What would motivate you to create time to focus on the diet? Check out the section in chapter five of this book about balance, and see what things in your life are draining your energy and need to be taken off your plate. Perhaps you need stronger boundaries and an ability to say no a little more often in service of yourself and your family.

4. "I am doing it about 90 percent, but that last 10 percent just feels like too much! Does a little bit here and there really matter?"

You bet it does! I have loads of stories where that last 10 percent made the difference in most of the symptoms going away. Honor yourself and do it perfectly—no excuses, no exceptions. Follow the ideas in this book, and find strategies for all the places that feel difficult. I know perfect sounds challenging, but once you have all the recipes collected and the meals figured out, you will be fine. That extra 10 percent is often the difference between completely eliminating a symptom and having it continue to be a problem.

5. "Remind me again why I am doing this. Will it really make that much of a difference to my son's life down the road? Convince me!"

My website (*www.foodsensitivechildren.com*) contains testimonials from some of the hundreds of families whose health, behavior, and learning have been positively impacted by changes in their diets. In the end, however, it is for you to find your own motivation. What means so much to you that you would be willing to make this "diet" a healthy way of living, instead? How might your life or the life of your son be impacted if his symptoms disappeared? Close your eyes, and picture your son crossing the stage at his high school graduation. What might you be feeling? What do you want to celebrate about the job you did as a parent in supporting him to get to that day? What kind of a parent do you want to be? What do you need to change now to make that happen? Chapter five contains several sections to help you increase your motivation to make successful changes in your life that will support your entire family.

6. "I need help, but I have no idea who to ask. Everyone else seems to be intimidated by the idea, and they can't seem to figure out how they might help. I have done okay with the basics at the start but now I feel I need some support to do this over the long term."

Having adequate help and support as you make these changes is very important. There is a section in chapter five of this book intended to help you clarify what type of help you most need and to notice how willing you are to ask for it. People are often intimidated by the idea of baking an egg-free, dairy-free, or gluten-free cake and need a little help to learn how. Give them a recipe, give them some of your flour mix or milk substitute, and perhaps even invite them over to do it with you. If the people in your life are still unwilling to give it a try, ask for help in other ways. Perhaps they could watch the kids while you grocery shop in peace or give you a break so you could get some exercise to help you decrease your stress. Be sure to care for yourself as you care for your family because if you are overwhelmed and stressed, the job seems much harder.

7. "I need new recipes! My kids hate what I am making, and it is discouraging."

The best recipes are the ones that create the comfort foods your kids are used to eating all the time. Check out the section at the back of the book with alternatives, and do your best to simply replace the ingredient you are avoiding in the recipe. If this isn't working well, I suggest you search for what you are looking for on the Internet. You will be amazed at the hundreds of recipes that will appear. Be sure it is a reputable website and that the recipes have been perfected so you don't waste a lot of ingredients. Check out the section in chapter six of this book that offers meal ideas for kids of all ages. Perhaps there are things here that will help. The resource section at the end of this book also contains loads of cookbooks and websites that offer recipe ideas.

8. "My response to this diet is all over the map! One minute, I embrace it, and another minute, I am throwing up my hands in despair over the work and time it takes. I get angry at the situation for a while, and then I am hopeful that it will make a big difference in our son's symptoms. I feel like I am on an emotional roller coaster."

Welcome to the experience of grief and loss related to diet change. It is an emotional journey with many ups and downs. Some days, things seem easy, and other days, you long to throw in the towel. Take a few minutes to read chapter four on resistance, change, grief and loss. It is common to be angry one minute, depressed over the topic another, and then connected to the hope and benefits of the diet after that. Offer yourself lots of grace for your journey, and know that all the responses are normal. Slowly but surely, you will gradually embrace the changes. Instead of being part of a "diet," your food choices will simply be your life choices. The benefits will become clear, and these will make the extra time and effort worth it. Some days, you will still hate it, and so will your child. Take a few minutes to notice how you are feeling, and then go and do something fun. Treat yourself to something you can eat that feels special, and remember how far you have come.

9. "How long does my son have to be on this diet? I don't think I can do it forever."

There is no easy answer to this question, as it depends on many things. If your son has a very serious problem with his trigger food, it is likely it will be at least some degree of an issue for the rest of his life. I'm sorry to have to tell you that! Your child may be able to tolerate very small amounts at times when his life is calm and relaxed. Food intolerances are impacted by our overall health and life experiences, so it is never a wise thing to challenge a food with your child when he is sick, tired, or stressed. The truth is that if your child's health improves, you will find the motivation to stay on the diet. You will grieve the loss, be angry, and bargain around the topic for a while, but eventually, it will become a part of your normal life. The long term benefits will be worth it.

Issues Related to Pregnancy, Breast Feeding, and Babies

1. "I am breastfeeding, my two month old son is constantly screaming, has green poop instead of golden yellow and I am absolutely exhausted! Is it possible that something I am eating is the problem? How would I ever figure out what food it might be?"

This is an amazingly common story! Yes, it is entirely possible—and even likely—that it is a food you are eating that is making your baby scream all the time. Please be sure, however, that you take your baby to the doctor for a complete check-up to rule out any other serious illnesses. The food to remove can be determined by completing the questionnaire in chapter three of this book. It is likely that the food bothering your baby is one you crave, eat almost every day, and has been a favorite of yours since childhood. When you are tired, your milk supply also diminishes, so it is important that you try and find ways to get a little more rest. If you can get someone to take your baby outside for a walk now and then, you will sleep better when you can't hear him fussing. Don't give in and start your baby on formula of any kind, if at all possible. If your child has colic, it is more likely he will react to milk-based formulas, and your problems will continue or get even worse. Also, over half the colicky babies bothered by dairy are also bothered by soya formula so do your best to continue to breast feed and adjust your own diet, instead.

2. "My baby is screaming all the time, and I have already removed the milk in my diet!"

How frustrating! First of all, reread the list of words in chapter six of this book that indicate the presence of dairy in foods. It is possible that you have missed something in your diet. Remember that to get the full benefit, you must remove 100 percent of all dairy-containing foods from your diet. Fill up with other delicious foods, and satisfy your craving with wonderful flavours of soya, rice, or coconut ice cream, but don't give in. If you are already doing the diet perfectly, look for another food by completing the questionnaire in chapter three of this book. What food are you consuming every day, and what food do you crave? What food do you most not want to give up? Be honest with yourself! You might find it helpful to keep a food diary to notice any correlation between your baby's symptoms and what you have eaten.

3. "I am pregnant and have heard that if I avoid foods that are a problem for me, it will decrease the chance that our child will be bothered. Should I change my diet now, and how will I know which food to remove?"

It is essential during pregnancy and when you are nursing that you eat a balanced, varied, and healthy diet. If a particular food seems to be causing symptoms, it is okay to remove it, as long as you replace it with a healthy alternative. If you remove oranges, for example, ensure you eat another food that is a good source of vitamin C. If you remove dairy products, talk to your doctor about adding a calcium supplement, and drink another type of milk, such as soya, rice, or almond, that is fortified with calcium. If your baby has recurrent hiccups while still in utero, this may indicate that something you are eating is bothering it so do a little detective work to see if you can find the culprit. Also, ensure you have removed any food that has been a problem for you in the past.

Situations Involving Other Methods of Testing

1. "I asked my pediatrician to refer our daughter to an allergist to see if we could do something to make her feel better. She is tired all the time, has stomach aches, wets the bed at the age of eight, and is crabby and uncooperative. He made the referral, and we saw the allergist last week. The allergist did extensive scratch tests on our daughter for a wide variety of foods and announced that she wasn't bothered by any of them. She tested positive for a couple of pollens and house dust, but nothing that is in season right now. He suggested I strip her bedroom and remove the carpet and all her stuffed animals, and when she heard what he said, she burst into tears. He offered to have me try an elimination diet with her, but I can't face the idea, as she hardly eats anything as it is. What can I do now?"

Your daughter's situation is a common one. Most reactions to food are not allergies, but intolerances which cannot be identified by any type of scratch testing. There is more information on this in chapter two. Elimination diets may be helpful, but many families find them impossible to do, because their children either refuse to eat the allowed foods or the parents don't feel they have enough information on how to do it and still feed the rest of their family. Sensitivity to house dust is very common and often improves dramatically when an offending food is removed from the diet. It is worth a try to adjust your daughter's diet before you remove all of her favorite stuffed animals and the carpet. I suggest you follow the process in chapter three of this book and identify the trigger food that may be the underlying cause for your daughter's symptoms. By removing only one food, the task is usually more manageable, and your chance of making a quick and dramatic improvement in her health is high. The rest of the book leads you, step by step, through a process to successfully adjust your daughter's diet.

2. "The naturopath has done some blood tests for food sensitivities and has told me to remove fifteen foods from our son's diet. That leaves me nothing to feed him! It is impossible."

This is an all-too-common story, and most parents have the same reaction that you have had. Removing that number of foods from your family's diet does make it feel impossible to find anything to cook. I encourage you to follow the process in chapter three of this book to identify the trigger food that is likely the cause of your child's symptoms. By removing the trigger food, most symptoms dramatically improve. It is also important to rotate the remaining foods so that they are not eaten any more often than every four days. This will decrease your son's exposure to secondary foods that may be a problem and allow his body to heal without removing them completely. It also is a healthy way for all children to eat, as they need a variety of nutrients.

Special Support for Grandparents and Teachers Who Want To Help

1. "I am a grandmother, and I know my daughter needs to change the diet of my grandchildren, but she refuses. I am afraid of

what is ahead for them if she doesn't. She says she is too busy and doesn't believe it will help. What can I do?"

I, too, am a grandmother and empathize with your situation. It is difficult to watch your grandchild be bothered by something you are quite sure has an easy solution. Do you remember being a young mom, trying your very best to do what is right for your child? Remember how you reacted when someone else tried to tell you what to do? Yup, I remember, too. All you can do is love your daughter and your grandchildren the best way you can. Serve them only healthy food at your house, and tell your daughter that you are committed to making your house a fun and healthy place to visit. Do it in a kind and supportive way, and teach your grandchildren how to eat and cook when they visit. Don't ever criticize their parents to them. Simply make your home a place they love to visit. It is okay to say the odd thing to your daughter here and there, but she will likely hear you better if you just accept and love her kids rather than try and tell her what to do. Perhaps you can buy a copy of this book and just leave it lying around. Trust that if and when her children's symptoms increase, she may be more motivated to change and listen to what you have to say.

2. "I am a teacher and see several kids in my class with health, behavior, or learning challenges that I think might benefit from addressing their foods. How can I approach the topic with a parent and not offend them?"

As you no doubt have already discovered, parents are very sensitive to criticism about their children. Tread lightly. The best way I have found is to encourage your parent's group to offer an evening workshop for families on the topic of food sensitivities and then encourage all your classroom parents to go. This topic, unfortunately, is still somewhat new and controversial, despite the wide range of credible evidence on the power of food on learning and behavior as well as health. My website contains lots of non-threatening information that might plant the seed and encourage them to explore the idea further. It is easier to encourage parents to seek medical help for health-related issues, and I wouldn't hesitate at all to encourage them seek help for issues that are a challenge for you in the classroom. Parents also value hearing all the positive things you have to say about their children and where their parenting strategies are being successful. Particularly if their child is difficult, they may have heard dozens and dozens of criticisms about them, so offer positive feedback on how you see their child. I'm not suggesting you make them up just to be nice. Make them real and honest examples of places where you know their child is amazing. You will win them over easily, and they may then be more willing to hear other ideas you might have for their child.

Supporting Children with Autism, Learning Disabilities and Other Challenges

1. "My child has autism, and there is much talk everywhere about the fact that the diet will help. I know people who swear by it, but I can't imagine trying it. Our son is so sensitive to textures and tastes, he hardly eats anything now."

Autism certainly adds extra challenges and work to your already busy life. I admire you for even asking the question and trying to explore the topic of food sensitivities for yourself. I have written an entire section on autism in this book because many families are considering adjusting the diet of their kids to see if it will make any difference in their symptoms. My first advice here is to carefully take time to look at the balance of your life. How many things are on your already full plate? Is there room for one more thing? I know there is great pressure on parents of kids with autism to try every therapy out there, and the cost and investment of time is huge. I know that as a parent, you have a very good intuition about what works for your own child, and I encourage you to listen to it. Don't just buy into the story that you need to do it all, but carefully explore the alternatives, and decide for yourself. I have worked with some families who never have time for a meal together or time to even go to the park, as they spend every waking minute giving their child some type of therapy. Children also need free time just to be themselves, and all families need fun time together. Honor yourself, your family, and your son by making choices that *feel* right to you and not choices that are done because you believe that to really love your child, you must do it all.

I have, however, personally witnessed the dramatic improvement that diet change can have on children with autism. I have seen children who did not speak at all begin talking in complete sentences after three weeks on the diet. I encourage you to read chapter seven on autism and then consider finding room in your life to try it. Don't be swayed into doing the dairy-free/gluten-free diet or the specific carbohydrate diet first. Please consider trying my approach of identifying the trigger food specific to your own child as outlined in chapter three. This process is much easier and has a much high chance of success because it focuses on the needs of your own unique child.

2. "My son is struggling at school. His reading is already behind, and they want to put him in a special program. Will changing his diet actually make a difference?"

There are many reasons children struggle at school, and it is very wise to get some academic testing done so you really understand your son's challenges. Be sure to choose carefully who does the testing so the experience for your child doesn't focus on failure and frustration.

Adjusting your child's diet has a very good chance of making it easier for him to focus and retain what he is learning. I have worked with many, children whose learning has improved significantly when we removed the trigger food from their diet. For years, I volunteered with the Learning Disabilities Association of British Columbia, helping adults adjust their diets to address some of their challenges, and I saw many wonderful changes there, as well. I think it is important to do everything you can to support your child having a positive learning experience at school. Time and support invested early pay off in the years to come. Our goal as parents is to maximize the potential of our children, and supporting their learning is a big part of that. If he requires extra tutoring or educational support, be sure it is appropriate for your child, and listen to his thoughts about it, as well as to his teachers. Be sure the experience is as positive as possible. If you change his diet at the same time, you might well be able to help him retain more of what he has learned and experience success sooner than with other special programs alone.

CHAPTER 8 HIGHLIGHTS

QUICK SOLUTIONS TO COMMON SITUATIONS

- Whatever challenges and frustrations you are experiencing, know that they are normal. Everyone finds diet change challenging some of the time, so refer to the commonly asked questions in this section to find some quick and helpful answers.

- No matter what frustrations you experience, seek out the support you need, and don't give up. Your child deserves to realize his or her full potential. Giving a diet change the chance to work is the only way you will know if it will make a difference.

- If you experience criticism from others, read the section on the voice of your saboteur and boundaries in chapter five, and problem-solve ways you can stay committed and strong in your resolve to give the diet your best effort.

- Be gracious and patient with yourself if you slip up. You are human, and so is your child. Do your best, and if you fall off the wagon, get back on and renew your commitment to do it.

- The questions in this chapter are categorized under the following headings to make it easier for you to access the information you need.

  1. Dealing with challenges and resistance in yourself and your family
  2. Special occasion strategies
  3. Managing physical symptoms
  4. Coping with resistance from friends, coworkers, teachers and health care professionals
  5. Making the changes sustainable
  6. Issues related to pregnancy, nursing and babies
  7. Situations involving other methods of testing

8. Special support for grandparents and teachers who want to help
9. Supporting children with autism, learning disabilities and other challenges.

EPILOGUE

MY PERSONAL STORY OF HOPE

"Hope is the anchor of the soul" (Hebrews 6:19)

It's been said that finding gifts in the adversities of our lives and using them to make a difference in the lives of others offers healing. My personal story is a testament to that wisdom. I share my story in the hope it will inspire you to consider altering your diet or that of someone you love to regain the health and joy that is possible for us all.

My health problems began in infancy, just as those of many of my clients. I was adopted as a baby, and the history that was available from my birth mother was sketchy at best. I was bottle-fed as an infant, and although I thrived, this was possibly the origin of the bowel inflammation that caused my symptoms years later. I had severe diaper rash as a baby and had my tonsils out at the age of four, which I know now, can be early indications of food sensitivities. The intolerances for certain foods that we inherit at birth play a significant role in determining our future health. Many children are intolerant to cow's milk, and this can be the primary cause of many childhood illnesses.

I was a healthy, happy toddler, and in my early school years, I was an active, bright little girl who was filled with a zest for life. In about grade three or four, I began to have stomach aches that often woke me up at night and usually appeared when I was nervous, excited, or anxious.

The doctor decided that it was likely a "nervous stomach" and no treatment was offered. I shudder now as I recall never having been asked directly if I was nervous about anything in particular. If someone had asked, I would have shared with them that yes, I was anxious because my dad had a drinking problem. It was one of those hidden secrets that few people knew, and I learned early on not to share the story except with a few close friends. I wish someone had seen past my bright and sunny exterior and actually spent time with me alone to ask how I really was.

My digestive symptoms continued to worsen as life at home became more stressful so I was sent to a gastroenterologist in search of some answers. Despite suffering the indignity of colonoscopies and drinking chocolate-flavored barium for x-rays, the doctors were unable to find a cause for my symptoms. A couple of years later, however, my dad courageously stopped drinking and my stomach aches became less of an issue in my life. I was grateful that the stress I had experienced years before had decreased and my dad became the wonderful man I now remember. Both my dad and my mom were a constant source of support and encouragement to me and I thrived in my high school years. I participated in music, sports, and social activities of all kinds and lived in a neighborhood full of kids where we played kick-the-can and swam in our pool every summer evening. My life was full of people who loved me and who supported my entire family.

Despite my mom's commitment to feed us only healthy food, I continued to be bothered by occasional stomach aches and I also developed acne as a teenager. The dermatologist gave me large doses of antibiotics which I took for many months. These upset the balance of bacteria in my bowel and made my digestive complaints even worse. Both symptoms would appear unannounced at unwelcome times such as first dates or during exams. It is only now that I understand the reason. Food intolerances are connected to the circumstances of life. Unlike true allergies, in which a reaction usually occurs immediately, food intolerances appear at a variety of different times and in different forms, depending on our life experiences. If you imagine a barrel full of water, there is one last drop that sends the water flooding over the edge. My yet-to-be-discovered food intolerances resulted in me living with the level of water in my barrel close to the very top. Any small food challenge or difficult life circumstance caused my barrel to overflow, and my symptoms increased. Perhaps I would get yet another stomach ache, develop a cough that wouldn't go away, or look in the mirror and see a face with several unwanted zits. I was totally frustrated, as were my parents, and none of the many doctors I visited could offer any answers.

When I went to university to get my nursing degree, my health seemed to stabilize. I lived at home for the first two years and then moved to an apartment with a friend for the final three. I ate quite well, considering I was often cooking for myself, and my symptoms didn't get any worse. I did discover, however, that beer made my stomach aches return in full force, so drinking was something I rarely did. I now know that the reason for this is that beer contains a large amount of gluten and years later, I would discover that I was gluten intolerant. Despite the hard work of university, my life was fun and interesting, and I thrived in the environment as I fulfilled a lifelong dream of becoming a nurse.

In 1975, I married my husband, a medical student, and we began our life together. His very favorite foods were white bread with cheese, so we often had this as a late-night snack. It was all he often felt like eating when he came home after several days on call and was so exhausted he could barely keep his eyes open. An inherited predisposition for gluten and dairy intolerances coupled with a runaway lifestyle set us both up for trouble tolerating these foods. When they are not completely digested, dairy and gluten-containing foods produce by-products related to the narcotic family (like morphine). This explains the craving for these particular foods I saw in my husband and myself as well as what I notice in my clients. Sadly, however, I did not yet have the wisdom to understand what was going on. The extra bread and cheese in my diet created a resurgence of my stomach aches and I found that I was more tired than I ever remembered being. I chalked it up to being newly married.

Despite working opposite shifts and schedules, my husband and I began to think about having children a couple of years later. Our first son was born in 1978 and he was a beautiful, robust little boy who screamed from the minute he arrived. No amount of breast feeding would quiet him and I was beyond exhaustion. I was a pediatric nurse who had worked in the intensive care nursery. Shouldn't I be able to care for my own healthy baby, as my doctor assured me he was? I still remember going to the pediatrician when our son was three months old, and in between sobs, telling him I was going to die caring for this baby. My baby screamed day and night and slept for no more than about twenty minutes at a time. I walked, drove, rocked, paced, cuddled, and everything else I could think of, but nothing seemed to help. I felt powerless, hopeless, and completely inadequate as a mother.

The pediatrician's response to my struggle was the beginning of my journey of healing. He casually mentioned an article he had read that encouraged nursing mothers to stop eating dairy products if they had colicky babies. Upon this advice, I immediately stopped all the dairy products I was eating, and a miracle occurred. Our son stopped crying and began to laugh. He slept—and as a result, so did I.

My own stomach aches also seemed to disappear, although it was a few more years before I made the true connection for myself. Although I was feeling better and our son was thriving, I had to face other people's doubts and criticisms about my decision to stop consuming dairy products myself and to avoid giving them to our son. Many were sure that our son would grow up with crumbling bones and poor nutrition. Staying strong in my commitment to do what our son needed wasn't always easy, but I was committed to him having the best start in life—and besides, I needed the sleep!

When our daughter was born eighteen months after our son, she did not seem to have any of his food issues. She was quiet, calm, full of smiles, and a joy to breast feed. However, at the age of two, after her first dose of antibiotics for a sore throat, her behavior became difficult and she had tantrums over the smallest request. She was often too tired to walk even a block and suffered from tummy aches and bladder pains much of the time. Where did my sunny little girl go? Why had all the things I had learned with our first son not made a difference for her? I kept her off dairy products, but the symptoms did not seem to improve. It would be another year and a half before I figured it out.

In the midst of caring for these two young children, I had a gall bladder attack that resulted in surgery to remove it. Because my gall bladder was filled with stones, the doctors reassured me that this was the reason for my years of stomach aches. Finally, I had an answer! Unfortunately, about six months after my gall bladder was removed, my symptoms reappeared, and I was again subjected to a number of unpleasant tests. Yet again, no answers were found. I was put on a medication to improve my digestion and told that I could not have any more children, because this medication could cause birth defects. I eventually stopped the medication as it was not relieving my symptoms, and we were hoping to have another baby. This doctor also took my husband aside in the hallway of the hospital and told him that he thought my symptoms were related to the stress I was under due to his hours of work and my busy life at home. I was upset that a professional had, once again, decided I was stressed without discussing it with me directly. I believe that patients need to be treated with respect and that professionals need to take time to ask patients about all aspects of their life. Making inaccurate assumptions can rob the patient of the opportunity to get the support and help that they need. It is one of the many reasons I am now a life coach, and this respectful listening is something I am committed to offering to all of my clients.

Our next son was born three years later, and I was on the lookout for food issues with him because, like his older brother, he hiccupped in utero. During my pregnancy, I was often awakened in the middle of the night by his violent hiccups that made my entire abdomen bounce. I nursed him at birth and again removed dairy products from my diet. Despite my best efforts, he developed repeated ear infections and ended up with tubes in his ears at six months of age. We brought him home after surgery and discovered his hearing had been compromised when he was captivated by the ticking grandfather clock in our living room, having never heard it before.

What did I miss? Why did removing dairy products from his diet not have the same impact it had on his brother? Despite switching him to soya formula, his health continued to deteriorate, and soon gastrointestinal symptoms appeared. To make matters worse, once I weaned him and returned to drinking milk and eating cheese myself, all my own digestive symptoms returned. I went to an allergist, convinced I had finally found my answer. Based on my history and symptoms, he concluded that I had been bothered by dairy products for most of my life and that they were the cause of my childhood stomach aches. I left his office inspired that perhaps I had found an answer to my years of troubling symptoms.

Four months later, we moved to Toronto so that my husband could complete his final year of surgery training. I left Vancouver with much sadness, as I was leaving behind all my friends and family whose support I counted on. Nonetheless, as we drove all across the country with our three very small children, I was looking forward to three weeks together as a family. The kids approached the trip with a wide-eyed sense of adventure and loved exploring each new campground as we went. They still look back on the trip with fond memories. Our second son, however, began to have more gastrointestinal symptoms and was very unwell by the time we reached Toronto. He was investigated by the pediatrician and subjected to unpleasant tests, but no answer was found. Symptoms began to increase in our other two children, and I was more overwhelmed than ever. I had one son struggling with recurrent ear infections; a daughter suffering from tummy aches, fatigue, confusion, and irritability; and another son with digestive complains and hyperactivity that kept him up every night from 2:00 a.m. until 5:00 a.m. I can still remember sitting on the beds of our sleeping children and asking God what on earth had happened to my life. I had always longed to be a mom, but this was not how I imagined it would be. Was He really there, and did He care that I was sinking?

As a result of the lack of sleep, stress, and lack of support, I became very ill. My eyes became swollen, and I had stomach aches again. I sought the help of an allergist in Toronto and learned in a phone call from him that my blood work had shown some unusual illness with no definitive treatment—more questions with no answers!

Because we had very little money and no local family support, I had only a two-hour window each week for a break. The babysitter arrived, and I was free for two glorious hours. I usually went to a bookstore and treated myself to a book and then sat and read it over a peaceful lunch. At the end of my rope one afternoon, I walked into a bookstore, and as always, God had been listening to my prayers. As I scoured the shelves for just the right book, I noticed one glowing on the shelf high in one corner of the store. Was I hallucinating? Perhaps all the stress and fatigue had finally gotten to me. I hesitantly reached for the book and was immediately captivated by the title, *"Changing Your Child's Behavior Chemistry."* I bought it, and in my short lunch break, scanned my way through the entire book. I felt as though someone had written a book specifically about my own children. I raced home, made an appointment with the pediatrician, and insisted on a referral to an allergist.

I took our daughter first, as her symptoms were the most complicated, but was horrified by what took place. The doctor poked her with over twenty needles while she cried, "Why are you letting them do this to me, Mommy?" She was three and a half years old. Tears were running down my cheeks as I did what I thought was required in order to help her get well. At the end of the testing, the doctor announced that the results were only 50 percent accurate for food, and he wanted to place her on a multiple food elimination diet. I wish he had told me this before I subjected my little girl to this unpleasant experience! I now know better. Scratch tests certainly have their place to determine environmental allergens, but only a very few ever need to be done. True food allergies are very rare, and most food reactions are, in fact, food intolerances. The distinction is important because intolerances are the result of inflamed bowel walls and an imbalance in bowel bacteria and can't be diagnosed by traditional allergy skin testing.

I returned home from the allergist committed to finding the answer to the struggles and challenges of our children. I went to the library, checked out several books, and read voraciously as soon as the kids went to bed. I found some of the answers in those pages and changed their diets the following morning. I removed milk from everyone's diet, eggs from our daughter's diet, and wheat from the diet of our youngest son. Within two weeks, the changes were nothing short of miraculous—no more diarrhea. No more tummy aches. No more ear infections. No more fatigue and confusion. Our daughter became an inquisitive sponge and learned more in two weeks than I would ever have believed was possible. Our children were healthy, happy, and bright. Finally, they were well. As I completely removed dairy products from the house, it made a big difference in how I felt, as well. My stomach aches all but disappeared and I felt better than I had in years.

We returned to Vancouver a few months later, excited to be home. My husband began medical practice, and we bought our first house. I took the risk of getting pregnant again, certain that I knew exactly how to care for myself and our baby to avoid all the pitfalls I had experienced before. I turned out to be right. Our gorgeous little girl arrived in this world having had no hiccups in utero as I avoided milk and wheat during the entire pregnancy. I monitored what I ate as I breast fed and she never got sick—no ear or throat infections. No screaming. No green poop. No tummy aches. She was a delightful, happy baby who continues to have this disposition to this day. She was a reward for all that I had learned and a gift to show me what is possible if food sensitivity issues are addressed early in life.

As our children's health improved, I was ecstatic. Some days, I was run off my feet with the busy pace of all their activities, but they were well, and I loved it all. I was totally unprepared for what came next.

Without warning, when our youngest daughter was only four months old, I began to experience profuse, bloody diarrhea, and I was terrified. I had a four-month-old, a four-year-old, a seven-year-old, and an eight-year-old—what if I had bowel cancer? What if I had Crohn's Disease?

I was nursing my baby—what if she got sick? I went to the hospital, afraid of what I might find out.

The doctor discovered that I had an overwhelming E.coli infection from something I had eaten. I was bleeding, in extreme pain, engorged with milk (as I couldn't feed my baby), and feeling totally miserable. After two weeks in the hospital on isolation, I finally went home. I was drinking only diluted pineapple juice and afraid to eat solid food, but I was desperate to see my family. It was difficult to get better, because of the busy pace of my life, so ten months later, I took a much-needed vacation to stay with a friend in Toronto. I needed some sleep and a break.

As the months went on, I learned very quickly that certain foods created symptoms, and my diet became more and more restricted. I developed red spots on my thighs that corresponded with pains in my joints, and no medical professional could find the answer. My story was minimized and dismissed, and no one could offer any solutions. Most physicians refused to believe my observation that altering my diet had an impact on my symptoms. I was frustrated and discouraged. This time, it was my health that was the problem, and again, I had no answers.

Finally, after almost twenty years of medical appointments with seventeen specialists and dozens of tests, I have a diagnosis for my problem. I have an autoimmune disease that is the result of the E.coli infection I had twenty-four years ago. A new doctor appeared in my life through a number of what I view as divinely inspired coincidences, and she has offered me her listening ear and her medical wisdom. She suggested I take an immune suppressant drug which makes a huge difference in my symptoms. I am taking it—although reluctantly, because of the long-term side effects—and I am committed to being off it very soon. I continue to explore alternative ways of healing, and each new piece of learning improves my health. I have slowed the pace of my life down to one that makes room for daily contemplative prayer, time with friends and family, and plenty of room for healthy food and exercise.

I am also blessed to have friends and family who care and who offer safe places for me to share my frustrations. I have learned a lot because of my experience with my children and have adapted my diet to maximize my health. If it were not for the wisdom I acquired in my effort to help them, I would not have the health I have today. God's guidance that day in the bookstore has impacted both my life and the lives of my family ever since. I will be forever grateful.

The support I have received along this journey from my husband has been nothing short of amazing. He embraced all the new foods that appeared on our dinner table and ate them without complaint. He, too, loved watching our kids get well and was the strength and support I leaned on when I was lost or confused about what to do next. He wholeheartedly supported our decision for me to be home and has worked long hours to make it all possible. Our marriage is a blessing we both treasure, and when we face the challenges of life, we work as a team to find creative answers and search for the next idea to try. Our commitment to each other and to our family is always what keeps us going.

The changes I made in the diet of my family occurred over twenty-five years ago and have been worth every minute of extra baking and creative meal planning. I know without a doubt that their health challenges would have continued to worsen, and many of the opportunities they have had would not have been possible. I am grateful every day for God's intervention and care. It has been my pleasure and privilege for twenty-five years to share the story of our children and to encourage other parents to take the risk and remove offending trigger foods from their child's diet. The healing that has often been possible for their children usually surpasses their wildest expectations.

I have a purpose in sharing this story. The issue of food sensitivities is a common one, and there are thousands of children and adults whose health is impacted every day. As a nurse and life coach, I offer my support and encouragement to others as they attempt to overcome the hurdles I once faced. Whether their adversity is related to diet or occurs because of other challenges in their lives, it is my privilege to help them reconnect to their own resilience and strength. I support them to courageously pursue their dreams and to believe anything is possible. My business card reads, "Hope is the Anchor of the Soul," and I believe this to be true. This phrase guides my own life, my coaching, and my words in this book.

One of the best ways to heal a long and difficult story is to find meaning in it. I have found meaning by offering my experiences to others with the goal that they will find hope. It is clear to me that God has been walking beside me through this entire journey. He has offered me books, supportive people, opportunities, and much more just when I have needed it most. Some days I wish I had found the solutions sooner, and some days I wish I had more healing for myself, but most days, I am grateful for where I am. As I watch our son and daughter-in-law use what I have learned to maximize the health of our grandsons, I know it has all been worth it. Our grandsons are bright, fun-loving, and healthy little boys who are thriving on a gluten-free, dairy-free, soya-free diet. I admire their mom's courage and perseverance in carefully adjusting her diet during pregnancy and breast feeding to offer her sons the very best chance at a healthy start in life. As a result, our grandsons eat a wide variety of healthy food and are the picture of health. Since beginning the writing of this book, we have also been blessed by the addition of a new little granddaughter to our family. Our daughter carefully adjusted her diet during her pregnancy and avoids the trigger foods she knows bother her while she is breast feeding. She and her husband are reaping the benefits of their commitment to health and enjoying a peaceful and happy baby.

The joy I feel as I watch my children and grandchildren thrive is a priceless blessing. They have helped me find much healing in my own story. I feel a deep sense of gratitude to them, my husband, my friends, and the countless clients and families I've had the privilege of working with. I am deeply thankful for their presence in my life.

NOTES

1. "United States Obesity Trends". *Centre for Disease Control and Prevention.*
   www.cdc.gov/obesity/data/trends.html (accessed October 1, 2011)
2. Brenda Wilson N.D. and Leonard Smith M.D., *Gut Solutions.* (Clearwater, Florida: Renew Life Press and Information, 2003), 3.
3. Brenda Wilson N.D. and Leonard Smith M.D., *Gut Solutions.* (Clearwater, Florida: Renew Life Press and Information, 2003), 3.
4. Brenda Wilson N.D. and Leonard Smith M.D., *Gut Solutions.* (Clearwater, Florida: Renew Life Press and Information, 2003), 3.
5. Gary Thibodeau A. PhD., and Kevin T. Patton PhD., *The Human Body in Health and Disease.* (St. Louis, Missouri: Mosby Inc., 1997), 418
6. Gary Thibodeau A. PhD., and Kevin T. Patton PhD., *The Human Body in Health and Disease.* (St. Louis, Missouri: Mosby Inc., 1997), 419
7. Gary Thibodeau A. PhD., and Kevin T. Patton PhD. *The Human Body in Health and Disease.* (St. Louis, Missouri: Mosby Inc., 1997), 421
8. Gary Thibodeau A. PhD., and Kevin T. Patton PhD. *The Human Body in Health and Disease.* (St Louis, Missouri: Mosby Inc., 1997), 426

9. Gary Thibodeau A. PhD., and Kevin T. Patton PhD., *The Human Body in Health and Disease.* (St. Louis, Missouri: Mosby Inc., 1997), 42

10. Brenda Wilson N.D., C.T. *Renew Your Life: Improved Digestion Through Detoxification* (Clearwater, Florida: Renew Life Press and Information Services, 2002), 32

11. Gary Thibodeau A. PhD., and Kevin T. Patton, PhD., *The Human Body in Health and Disease.* (St. Louis, Missouri: Mosby Inc., 1997), 426

12. Gary Thibodeau A. PhD., and Kevin T. Patton, PhD. *The Human Body in Health and Disease.* (St. Louis, Missouri: Mosby Inc., 1997), 424

13. Janice M. Vickerstaff Joneja, PhD. R.D., *Dealing With Food Allergies in Babies and Children.* (Boulder, Colorado: Bull Publishing Company, 2007), 11

14. R. Bowen. "Fundamental Physiology and Anatomy of the Digestive System", *Colorado Hypertexts for Biomedical Sciences,* www.vivocolostate.edu/hbooks/pathphys (accessed October 1, 2011)

15. Natasha Campbell-McBride M.D. *Gut and Psychology Syndrome* (Soham, Cambridge: Medinform Publishing, 2004), 29

16. Brenda Wilson, N.D. and Leonard Smith M.D., Gut Solutions. (Clearwater, Florida: Renew Life Press and Information, 2003), 7

17. Natasha Campbell-McBride M.D. *Gut and Psychology Syndrome* (Soham, Cambridge: Medinform Publishing, 2004), 46

18. Janice M. Vickerstaff Joneja PhD. R.D. *Dealing With Food Allergies in Babies and Children.* (Boulder, Colorado: Bull Publishing Company, 2007), 2

19. Janice M. Vickerstaff Joneja, PhD. R.D. *Dealing With Food Allergies in Babies and Children.* (Boulder, Colorado: Bull Publishing Company, 2007), 3

20. Janice M. Vickerstaff Joneja PhD. R.D. *Dealing With Food Allergies in Babies and Children.* (Boulder, Colorado: Bull Publishing Company, 2007), 58

21. J. H. Elder, and others, "Review of the Gluten-Free, Casein-Free Diet in Autism: Results of a Preliminary Double Blind

Clinical Trial," *Journal of Autism and Development Disorders*, 36, (2006) 413-420.

22. Natasha Campbell-McBride. M.D., *Gut and Psychology Syndrome* (Soham, Cambridge: Medinform Publishing, 2004), 71

23. Orian C. Truss, M.D. *The Missing Diagnosis*. (Birmingham, Alabama, The Missing Diagnosis Incorporated, 1985), 63

24. Janice M. Vickerstaff Joneja PhD, R.D. "Dietary Management of Histamine Intolerance" www.allergynutrtion.com http:// www.allergynutrition.com/resources/FAQ/4/Histamine%20 intolerance.pdf (accessed October 1, 2011)

25. "Stages of Change Model" www.addictioninfo.org http:// www.addictioninfo.org/articles/11/1/Stages-of-Change-Model/Page1.html (accessed October 1, 2011)

26. Elizabeth Kubler-Ross MD. *On Death and Dying*. (New York, New York: Touchstone, 1969), 51

27. Laura Whitworth, Henry Kimsey-House, and Phil Sandahl, *Co-Active Coaching*. (Palo Alto, California: Davies-Black Publishing, 1998), 226

28. Laura Whitworth, Henry Kimsey-House, and Phil Sandah,. *Co-Active Coaching*. (Palo Alto, California: Davies-Black Publishing, 1998), 182

29. Laura Whitworth, Henry Kimsey-House, and Phil Sandahl, *Co-Active Coaching*. (Palo Alto, California: Davies-Black Publishing, 1998), 25

30. "The Power of Accountability" www.coachville.com (accessed April 15, 2009)

31. Gordon Neufeld Ph.D., and Gabor Mate M.D., *Hold Onto Your Kids: Why Parents Need To Matter More Than Peers*. (Toronto, Ontario: Vintage Canada, 2005), entire book

32. Gordon Neufeld Ph.D., and Gabor Mate M.D. *Hold Onto Your Kids: Why Parents Need To Matter More Than Peers*. (Toronto, Ontario: Vintage Canada, 2005), 59

33. Bette Hagman. *The Gluten-Free Gourmet Bakes Bread*. (New York, New York: Henry Holt and Company LLC, 1999) entire book

34. Janice M. Vickerstaff Joneja PhD. R.D. *Dealing With Food Allergies in Babies and Children*. (Boulder, Colorado: Bull Publishing Company, 2007), 306

35. Natasha Campbell-McBride M.D. *Gut and Psychology Syndrome* (Soham, Cambridge: Medinform Publishing, 2004), 25

36. Janice M. Vickerstaff Joneja PhD. R.D. *Dealing With Food Allergies in Babies and Children*. (Boulder, Colorado: Bull Publishing Company, 2007), 306

37. Janice M. Vickerstaff Joneja PhD. R.D. *Dealing With Food Allergies in Babies and Children*. (Boulder, Colorado: Bull Publishing Company, 2007), 307

38. Janice M. Vickerstaff Joneja PhD. R.D. *Dealing With Food Allergies in Babies and Children*. (Boulder, Colorado: Bull Publishing Company, 2007), 308

39. Janice M. Vickerstaff Joneja PhD. R.D. *Dealing With Food Allergies in Babies and Children*. (Boulder, Colorado: Bull Publishing Company, 2007), 308

40. "Prevalence of Autism in Canada" www.autismsocietycanada.ca http://www.autismsocietycanada.ca/index.php?option=com_content&view=article&id=55&Itemid=85&lang=en (accessed October 1, 2011)

41. Gordon Neufeld Ph.D., and Gabor Mate M.D. *Hold Onto Your Kids: Why Parents Need To Matter More Than Peers*. (Toronto, Ontario: Vintage Canada, 2005), 256

42. Brene Brown. Ph.D., L.M.S.W. *I Thought It Was Just Me: Women Reclaiming Power and Courage in a Culture of Shame*. (New York, New York: Penguin Group, 2007), entire book

43. Pema, Chodrun, *Taking The Leap-Freeing Ourselves from Old Habits and Fears*. (Boston, Massachusetts:Shambala Publications, 2009), 15

BIBLIOGRAPHY
AND RESOURCES

BOOKS

Barnard, Neal M.D. *Breaking the Food Seduction*. New York, New York: St. Martin's Press, 2003

Bateson-Koch D.C., N.D. *Allergies: Disease in Disguise*. Summertown, Tennessee: Books Alive, 1994

Braly, James M.D., and Hoggan, Ron M.A. *Dangerous Grains*. New York, New York: Penguin Putnam Inc., 2002

Breneman, James. *Handbook of Food Allergies*. New York, New York: Marcel Dekker, Inc. 1987

Brown, Brene Ph.D., L.M.S.W. *The Gifts of Imperfection*. Center City, Minnesota: Hazelden, 2010.

Brown, Brene Ph.D., L.M.S.W. *I Thought It Was Just Me: Women Reclaiming Power and Courage in a Culture of Shame*. New York, New York: Penguin Group, 2007.

Campbell, T. Colin PhD, and Campbell, Thomas M. *The China Study*. Dallas, Texas: Benbella Books, 2006

Campbell-McBride, Natasha M.D. *Gut and Psychology Syndrome*. Soham, Cambridge: Medinform Publishing, 2004

Chodron, Pema. *Taking the Leap—Freeing Ourselves from Old Habits and Fears*. Boston, Massachusetts: Shambhala Publications, 2009

Cloud, Dr. Henry, and Townsend, Dr. John. *Boundaries: When to Say YES When to Say No to Take Control Of*

Your Life. Grand Rapids, Michigan: Zondervan Publishing House, 1992

Elder, J. H. and others, "Review of the Gluten-Free, Casein-Free Diet in Autism: Results of a Preliminary Double Blind Clinical Trial," *Journal of Autism and Development Disorders,* 36, 2006

Ernsperger, Lori Ph.D., Stegen-Hanson, Tania OTR/L. *Just Take A Bite: Easy, Effective Answers to Food Aversions and Eating Challenges.* Arlington, Texas: Future Horizons Inc., 2004

Feingold, Ben F. M.D. *Why Your Child is Hyperactive.* Toronto, Ontario: Random House Inc., 1975

Friedman, Marilyn PhD., M.S., M.A., R.N., Bowden, Vicky R. D.N.Sc., R.N., and Jones, Elaine Ph.D, M.S., R.N. *Family Nursing: Research, Theory, and Practice.* Upper Saddle River, New Jersey: Pearson Education Inc., 2003

Fuhrman, Joel M.D. *Disease Proof Your Child.* New York, New York: Martin's Press, 2005

Gottschall, Elaine. B.A., M.Sc. *Breaking the Vicious Cycle.* Baltimore, Ontario: Kirkton Press Ltd., 2004

Hersey, Jane. *Why Can't My Child Behave?* Williamsburg, Virginia: Pear Tree Press Inc., 2006

Hister, Art. *Guide to Living a Long and Healthy Life.* Vancouver, British Columbia: Greystone Books, 2003

Joneja, Janice M. Vickerstaff PhD., R.D. *Dealing with Food Allergies: A Practical Guide to Detecting Culprit Foods and Eating a Healthy, Enjoyable Diet.* Boulder, Colorado: Bull Publishing, 2003

Joneja, Janice M. Vickerstaff. PhD., R.D. *Dealing With Food Allergies in Babies and Children.* Boulder, Colorado: Bull Publishing Company, 2007

Katie, Byron. *Who Would You Be Without Your Story?* Carlsbad, California: Hay House Inc, 2008

Kennedy, Diane M. *The ADHD Autism Connection.* Colorado Springs, Colorado: Waterbrook Press, 2002

Kubler-Ross, Elisabeth MD. *On Death and Dying.* New York, New York: Touchstone, 1969

Levinson, Harold N. M.D. *Smart But Feeling Dumb: The Challenging New Research On Dyslexia—And How It May Help You.* New York, New York: Warner Books Inc., 1994

Mate, Gabor M.D. *Scattered Minds: A New Look At The Origins and Healing of Attention Deficit Disorder.* Toronto, Ontario: Vintage Canada, 2000

Mate, Gabor M.D. *When The Body Says No: The Cost of Hidden Stress.* Toronto, Ontario: Vintage Canada, 2004

McCarthy, Jenny. *Louder Than Words: A Mother's Journey in Healing Autism.* New York, New York: Penguin Group, 2007

McCarthy, Jenny. *Mother Warriors.* New York, New York: Penguin Group (USA) Inc., 2008

Neufeld, Gordon Ph.D., and Mate, Gabor M.D. *Hold Onto Your Kids: Why Parents Need To Matter More Than Peers.* Toronto, Ontario: Vintage Canada, 2005

Pescatore, Fred MD. *The Allergy and Asthma Cure.* Hoboken, New Jersey: John Wiley and Sons, 2003

Rapp, Doris M.D. *Is This Your Child: Discovering and Treating Unrecognized Allergies in Children and Adults.* New York, New York: William Morrow and Company Inc., 1991

Rapp, Doris M.D. *Allergies and Your Family.* New York, New York: Sterling Publishing, 1980

Rice, Phillip L. *Stress and Health.* Pacific Grove, California: Brooks/Cole Publishing Company, 1999

Shulman, Dr.Joey. *Winning the Food Fight.* Mississauga, Ontario: John Wiley and Sons, 2003

Smith, Lendon H. M.D. *Improving Your Child's Behavior Chemistry.* Englewood Cliffs, New Jersey: Prentice-Hall Inc., 1984

Thibodeau, Gary A. PhD., and Patton, Kevin T. PhD. *The Human Body in Health and Disease.* St. Louis, Missouri: Mosby Inc., 1997

Truss, C. Orian M.D., *The Missing Diagnosis.* Birmingham, Alabama, The Missing Diagnosis Incorporated, 1985.

Whitworth, Laura, Kimsey-House, Henry, and Sandahl, Phil. *Co-Active Coaching.* Palo Alto, California: Davies-Black Publishing, 1998

Wilson, Brenda N.D., and Smith, Leonard M.D. *Gut Solutions*. Clearwater, Florida: Renew Life Press and
Information Services, 2003

Wilson, Brenda N.D., C.T. *Renew Your Life: Improved Digestion Through Detoxification*. Clearwater, Florida: Renew Life Press and Information Services, 2002

Wilson, James L. N.D., D.C., Ph.D. *Adrenal Fatigue*. Petalulma, California: Smart Publications, 2007

Wong, Donna L. PhD., R.N., PNP., CPN, FAAN. *Nursing Care of Infants and Children*. St. Louis, Missouri: Mosby Inc., 1999

Yapko, Diane. *Understanding Autism Spectrum Disorders*. New York, New York: Jessica
Kingsley Publishers Ltd, 2003

WEBSITES

The Internet has made it much easier to access resources on topics of all kinds. There are new websites being added almost daily so it is worth doing an Internet search often to see what new resources have been developed. It is important, however, that you discuss any issues related to your health with competent health care practitioners and investigate the credibility of the information you are reading. This list is offered only as a brief sampling of some of the websites I have found helpful. I use the Internet often for everything from finding a specific recipe to searching for health related information.

GLUTEN—FREE DIET INFORMATION

www.americanceliac.org
This website has been developed by the American Celiac Disease Alliance and has information on links to other diseases often related to gluten intolerance.

www.celiac.ca
This is the official website of the Canadian Celiac Association. It contains information on most topics related to gluten intolerance and has an

online store that sells a wide range of pocket guides and resources. It also lists all the local chapters and support groups throughout Canada.

www.celiac.com
This website discuses the physiology of celiac disease and is a good resource for all the foods that contain gluten.

www.foodphilosopher.com
This is a website with good information on gluten-free living as well as recipes. The authors have also written a number of cookbooks for gluten-free diets including the *Gluten-free for Good Health Cookbook* and *Gluten-free Baking Classics* which can be ordered on their website.

www.glutenfreechecklist.com
This is a site that has taken the time to investigate all the best gluten-free products on the market and evaluate them. Membership to this site is free.

www.glutenfreegirl.com
This is a website written by a woman who experienced years and years of illness before being diagnosed with celiac disease. She is also a writer so this website is loaded with her own experiences and perspectives as well as fabulous recipes. She is married to a chef and has a little girl of her own.

www.gflinks.com
This is a website that is loaded with links and resources related to gluten-free living.

www.glutenfreerestaurants.org
This website allows you to search for restaurants in the United States that offer gluten-free meals. The gluten-free restaurant program is run by the Gluten Intolerance Group of North America. Unfortunately it does not offer the same service for Canadian restaurants but it is helpful if you are travelling to the United States.

GLUTEN—FREE, CASEIN—FREE DIET

www.gfcfdiet.com
This is a comprehensive resource for families wanting to try the gluten-free casein free diet. It is geared towards parents with an autistic child and offers forums for parents to share their experiences.

DAIRY—FREE DIET INFORMATION

www.godairyfree.org
A comprehensive resource that offers ideas and support for lactose free, casein free and milk free diets. The website includes a list of suggested books along with cooking hints and recipe ideas.

FOOD ALLERGY RESOURCES

www.aaia.ca
This is the website of the Allergy and Asthma Information Association. This is an organization committed to improving the quality of life for Canadians affected by allergies, asthma and anaphylaxis. They focus on education and prevention and their website has a section on how to manage your child's food sensitivities at school.

www.allergynutrition.com
This is the website of Dr. Janice Vickerstaff Joneja. She is a registered dietician who also has a Ph.D in medical microbiology and immunology. She is the author of *Dealing with Food Allergies in Babies and Children* as well as a number of other books on nutrition. Her website contains reference materials on many aspects of food sensitivities and the low histamine diet.

www.anaphylaxis.org
This is the website of Anaphylaxis Canada with accurate information and products you can order to educate people on food allergies. They sell excellent teaching tools for the use of an Epi pen and ingredient cards you can take to the grocery store and restaurants to ensure you

avoid the offending trigger foods. This website also contains many great children's books with stories of characters dealing with a wide variety of food allergies as well as resources to help you educate your child's school.

www.calgaryallergy.ca
This website offers a comprehensive list of all the food families. Although a reaction to one food in a family does not guarantee a reaction to the others, in a small child it is wise to delay addition of other foods in the same family as the one that they react to. This website also contains a wealth of articles on many issues related to food sensitivities as well as chemicals and inhalants

www.histame.com
This is the website of the company that manufactures Histame, a supplement that can be helpful if your child is bothered by the histamine in foods. It contains a list of symptoms as well as a detailed list identifying foods that contain large amounts of histamine. For a more complete explanation of this diet, refer to Dr. Janice Vickerstaff Joneja's website at *www.allergynutrition.com.*

www.kidswithfoodallergies.org
This website is the largest online support network for parents managing children with food allergies. It offers a free associate membership that allows access to many resources and their on-line support groups. A family membership for $25 per year also allows access to their online resources and their bank of over 1200 food allergy specific recipes.

www.livingwithout.com
This is an outstanding website that offers daily recipes and many hints and ideas for dealing with food sensitivities in children. They also publish a magazine that is well worth getting as the recipes are always delicious and most are kid friendly. The magazine also contains helpful and informative articles related to food sensitivities in children.

HEALTH AND ILLNESS IN CHILDREN AND ADULTS

www.diseaseproof.com
This is the blog of Dr Joel Fuhrman M.D. where he posts articles related to children and health.

www.doctoroz.com
This is the website of Dr. Oz, the cardiac surgeon who has his own medical TV show. It offers accurate information on a wide range of topics and medical conditions. You can search for a topic and find a number of resources, including short videos. There are many resources related to the health and diet of children.

www.drfuhrman.com
Dr. Joel Fuhrman M.D. is the author of the book *Disease-Proof Your Child*. The book, as well as his website, offers compelling statistics about the preventative benefits of feeding your child well. He discusses how a nutritionally sound diet rich with fruits, vegetables, nuts, seeds, and legumes can help you child prevent many adult diseases as they grow older. His website offers a number of a different membership options that enable you to access his teleconferences and other resources.

www.thelearningcommunity.us
This is a website written by professionals on the health, learning, and behavior of children. There are resources for children from babies to adolescents and a large selection of great videos on topics that affect children and their families.

www.vivo.colostate.edu/hbooks/index.html
A website from Colorado State college that has a wide variety of online textbooks on topics related to pathophysiology and other medical topics.

PREGNANCY AND BREAST FEEDING

www.circleofmoms.com
This is a community with resources offered by moms for moms. You can post a question and then listen to the responses and experiences of other moms or you can join a community of moms with challenges or situations similar to yours. There are many communities on this website related to food sensitivities and how to manage children with these challenges.

www.kellymom.com
This is a popular website that offers evidence based information on pregnancy, infant sleep, and breast feeding. It is written by a Board Certified Lactation Consultant and contains comprehensive, accurate information.

AUTISM

www.autismndi.com
This is a website devoted to parents attempting a gluten-free and dairy-free diet to support their child with autism. There is a list of resources and professionals offering information on this diet as well as a directory of volunteers willing to help parents make the necessary changes. This website also contains a comprehensive list of research and articles related to diet, digestive health, and autism which may be printed off and taken to your doctor to support your belief that removal of trigger foods has made a difference in your child.

www.autismspeaks.org
This website was started in 2005 by grandparents of a child with autism. They are committed to raising funds for research, raising awareness of the disease, and advocating for families. The site has many scientific links on the current medical research related to autism and has over 236,000 fans on their Facebook page.

www.autismsupportnetwork.com

This comprehensive website offers free support groups and links to access local support in your own community. Their mission is to connect, guide, and unite and their goal is to help parents to find support and eliminate the need to reinvent the wheel or go it alone.

www.autismtoday.com

This website contains an extensive list of conferences related to autism held throughout North America as well as a wide variety of online and teleconference courses. It has over 5000 articles and links to professionals and resources throughout Canada and the United States.

SPECIFIC CARBOHYDRATE DIET

www.breakingthevisciouscycle.info

This website discusses the specific carbohydrate diet that is often used to treat inflammatory bowel diseases and autism. Elaine Gottschall began her search for an answer when her four year old daughter was diagnosed with inflammatory bowel disease in the 1950's. No successful treatment could be found and her daughter's health was failing so she searched for answers herself. After years of research and the successful treatment of her daughter, Elaine Gottschall found that removing all grains and complex carbohydrates from the diet improved the symptoms significantly. The website supports her book *Breaking the Vicious Cycle*.

www.scdiet.org

This website offers a community of support and research based information on the specific carbohydrate diet. It also contains a comprehensive list of resources related to this diet and a section with personal stories of patients who are successfully implementing the diet.

PARENTING

www.cloudtownsend.com

This is the official website of Henry Cloud and John Townsend, the authors of the book entitled *Boundaries*. They are also the authors of numerous other successful books on relationships of all kinds. Their website is a wonderful resource for short, instructive videos on a wide range of topics. By searching for a topic or an age group, you can access short videos where the author's respond to questions they are commonly asked. There are many videos related to parenting children of all ages. This website has a Christian perspective on some of the topics.

www.educo.ca/adventureschool.php
This is the camp in 100 Mile House, British Columbia that has been so life changing for our family. Their willingness to adjust the diet of their campers while not making the child uncomfortable is in keeping with their respectful view on how they treat children. The camp offers a wide variety of outdoor experiences for kids and families of all ages in a rustic, mountain setting.

www.gordonneufeld.com
The website that offers on-line courses and information based on Dr. Neufeld's book *Hold onto Your Kids*. His book is a valuable resource for parents and discusses his theories related to attachment needs and children. His in person courses are highly sought after and are led by trained facilitators.

LEARNING DISABILITIES

www.ldac-acta.ca
This is the official website of the Learning Disabilities Association of Canada. It contains information about the definition of learning disabilities as well as links to the local associations in each province.

www.ldrc.ca
This website has an extensive resource list of learning disability services in Canada as well a number of testing materials to determine if your child has a learning disability. There is also access to special tutoring courses as well as information on helping your child cope both at home and at school.

www.ncld.org
This is a US based online resource that contains articles and information related to children of all ages with learning disabilities. These articles cover topics related to advocating for your child at school and supporting your child at home, as well as many articles that address the emotional impact of these challenges on children and their family.

CHANGE

www.addictioninfo.org
This is one of the best websites that discusses how the stages of change relate to addictions of all kinds. It emphasizes that change is a process and that progression through these stages is not necessarily linear. People must be motivated to change and, even then, they often slip and slide from one stage to another until they are able to achieve sustainable change.

RECIPE BOOKS

The books below offer dependable recipes that work well with a variety of substitutions. Even if the particular recipe does not suit exactly the substitutions you require, make the appropriate adjustment and give it a try. One of the best resources for recipes, however, is the Internet. If you search for the particular recipe you are looking for and include the foods you need to avoid, you will usually find dozens of recipes that will fit the bill. Be careful to read through the suggestions and pick recipes that come for reputable sources so that you can ensure they have been adequately tested. It is very frustrating and expensive to make an entire batch of cookies or a cake and have it flop completely. For recipes requiring gluten-free flour, the mix that has been listed in this book usually works well.

Bager, Jodi, and Lass Jenny. *Everyday Grain-Free Gourmet.* North Vancouver, Canada: Whitecap Books, 2008
Bager, Jodi, and Lass, Jenny. *Grain-Free Gourmet.* North Vancouver, Canada: Whitecap Books, 2005

Barnard, Tanya, and Kramer Sarah. *How It All Vegan*. Vancouver, Canada: Arsenal Pulp Press, 2003

Barnard, Tanya, and Kramer, Sarah. *The Garden of Vegan*. Vancouver, Canada: Arsenal Pulp Press, 2002

Burton, Dreena. *Eat, Drink, and Be Vegan*. Vancouver, Canada: Arsenal Pulp Press, 2008

Conrad, Kendall. *Eat Well Feel Well*. New York, New York: Clarkson Potter/Publishers, 2006

Hagman, Bette. *The Gluten-Free Gourmet Bakes Bread*. New York, New York: Henry Holt and Company LLC, 1999

Hagman, Bette. *The Gluten-Free Gourmet Cooks Comfort Foods*. New York, New York: Henry Holt and Company LLC, 2004

Hammond, Leslie, and Rominger, Lynne Marie. *Allergy Proof Recipes for Kids*. Beverly, Massachusetts: Fair Winds Press, 2003

McKenna, Erin. *Babycakes*. New York, New York: Clarkson Potter, 2009

Moskowitz, Isa Chandra, and Romero, Terry Hope. *Vegan CupcakesTake over the World*. Cambridge, Massachusetts: Da Capo Press, 2006

Nardone, Silvana. *Cooking for Isaiah*. United States: Readers Digest Association Inc, 2010.

O'Brien, Susan. *The Gluten-Free Vegan*. Philadelphia, Pennsylvania: Da Capo Press, 2007

Prasad, Raman. *Recipes for the Specific Carbohydrate Diet*. Beverly Massachusetts: Fair Winds Press, 2008

Roberts, Annalise G. *Gluten-Free Baking Classics*. Berkeley, California: Agate Publishing, 2008

Seinfeld, Jessica. *Deceptively Delicious*. New York, New York: Melcher Media, 2007

Washburn, Donna and Butt, Heather. *Complete Gluten-Free Cookbook*. Toronto, Ontario: Robert Rose Inc, 2007

INDEX

V

Values and motivation 119–125
Vega testing 54

W

Wheat substitution 181
White blood cells 31
Withdrawal 63, 67, 152–154, 157, 164,
    212, 229, 234

Y

Yeast 5, 13, 22, 40, 57, 58

CPSIA information can be obtained at www.ICGtesting.com
Printed in the USA
LVOW061856120612

285799LV00002B/270/P